DIFFERENTIAL DIAGNOSIS IN PATHOLOGY:
BREAST DISORDERS

DIFFERENTIAL DIAGNOSIS IN PATHOLOGY

Series Editor: JONATHAN I. EPSTEIN, M.D.

Urologic Disorders
Jonathan I. Epstein, M.D.

Liver Disorders
Swan N. Thung, M.D.
Michael A. Gerber, M.D.

Bone and Joint Disorders
Edward F. McCarthy, M.D.

Breast Disorders
Ayten Someren, M.D.
C. Whitaker Sewell, M.D.

DIFFERENTIAL DIAGNOSIS IN PATHOLOGY:
BREAST DISORDERS

AYTEN SOMEREN, M.D.

Professor
Department of Pathology and Laboratory Medicine
Emory University School of Medicine
Atlanta, Georgia

C. WHITAKER SEWELL, M.D.

Professor
Department of Pathology and Laboratory Medicine
Emory University School of Medicine
Atlanta, Georgia

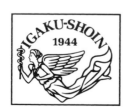

IGAKU-SHOIN   New York • Tokyo

Published and distributed by

IGAKU-SHOIN Medical Publishers, Inc.
One Madison Avenue, New York, New York 10010

IGAKU-SHOIN Ltd.,
5-24-3 Hongo, Bunkyo-ku, Tokyo 113-91.

Library of Congress Cataloging-in-Publication Data

Someren, Ayten.
    Differential diagnosis in pathology : breast disorders /
Ayten Someren, C. Whitaker Sewell.
        p.   cm.—(Differential diagnosis in pathology)
    Includes bibliographical references and index.
        1. Breast—Histopathology.   2. Breast—Diseases—
Diagnosis.   3. Diagnosis, Differential.   4. Breast—Biopsy.
I. Sewell, C. Whitaker.   II. Title.   III. Series.
        [DNLM: 1. Breast Diseases—diagnosis.   2. Breast
Diseases—pathology.   3. Diagnosis, Differential.
WP 840 S694d 1996]
RG493.S66   1996
618.1'9075—dc20
DNLM/DLC
for Library of Congress   96-3027
                                                                                                CIP

ISBN: 0-89640-314-9 (New York)
ISBN: 4-260-14314-X (Tokyo)

Printed and bound in the U.S.A.

10   9   8   7   6   5   4   3   2   1

PREFACE

Many current excellent books on general surgical pathology and recent textbooks and atlases devoted to breast disorders provide detailed coverage of the pathology of the breast. Although the differential diagnoses are included in these sources, they offer limited text and illustrations depicting differential diagnostic problems.

This book is designed to help the pathologist in the differential diagnosis of the more common lesions of the breast. It also brings to attention some of the less common lesions which may be overlooked or misdiagnosed. The book is divided into nine sections which cover those areas in breast pathology where the differential diagnostic problems commonly occur. The text in each section is divided into subsections which discuss the general considerations, clinical, imaging and gross features of the lesions, and histologic appearances. In discussion of the histologic characteristics, a comparative approach is used, with chapters designed to address the differential diagnostic problems. Emphasis is placed on detailed discussion of boundaries between lesions (hyperplastic vs. neoplastic, benign vs. malignant). The different viewpoints of experts in classification and terminology of various breast lesions is pre-sented. Some of the less well defined lesions are also briefly addressed. In the final brief chapter basic concepts of specimen radiograph interpretation are discussed and illustrated, to help the pathologist evaluate non-palpable, mammographically detected breast lesions.

The illustrations are selected to demonstrate the differential diagnostic features. In selection of illustrations, emphasis is placed on both low and high power microscopic observations, and application of immunohistochemical studies where appropriate. The ultrastructural findings are not emphasized. Large numbers of illustrations have been selected to thoroughly demonstrate the differential diagnostic points. The illustrations are discussed and referenced in the text and, therefore, figure legends are kept rather brief.

The bibliography is also brief, since this book is more of a guidebook than a textbook. Many of the classic references are included, as well as some of the more recent references that cover controversial areas.

We hope that the approach taken by this book will be helpful to the pathologist in the differential diagnosis of breast disorders, and will provide a practical and useful supplement to the existing texts on the subject.

DEDICATION

To our residents and students

ACKNOWLEDGMENTS

This book could not have been possible without the cumulative contributions of many, to whom we are grateful. Ms. Stephanie Cook, Ms. AnnaLee Boyett and Ms. Sandra Estep typed the entire manuscript and, together with Mr. Robert Santoianni, assisted us with their efforts during different stages of development of this book. Dr. Debra L. Monticciolo, Director, Division of Breast Imaging, Department of Radiology, Emory University School of Medicine allowed us to photograph specimen radiographs prepared by her department. They deserve special recognition.

The histopathologic sections from which the photographs are taken are largely the product of the histology laboratories at Emory University and Grady Memorial Hospitals. The black and white prints of the microscopic photographs are the work of the Medical Illustration Department at Emory University and Mr. Robert Santoianni of the Electron Microscopy Laboratory at Emory University Hospital. We extend our special thanks to all of these individuals for their skilful contributions.

We are indebted to the staff of Igaku-Shoin Medical Publishers for their interest and cooperation in all stages of development of this book. Ms. Lila Maron, Vice President, Editorial, and Ms. Gita Bhattacharji, Production Supervisor, deserve special thanks for their support.

CONTENTS

SECTION 1: ADENOSIS

1 Sclerosing Adenosis vs Tubular Carcinoma **2**

2 Perineural Space Extension in Sclerosing Adenosis vs Perineural Invasion by Infiltrating Carcinoma **6**

3 Nonneoplastic Apocrine Alterations in Sclerosing Adenosis vs Apocrine Carcinoma **8**

4 Sclerosing Adenosis with Marked Ductular Attenuation vs Infiltrating Lobular Carcinoma **12**

5 Microglandular Adenosis vs Tubular Carcinoma **14**

6 Sclerosing Adenosis vs Radial Scars and Complex Sclerosing Lesions (Radial Sclerosing Lesions) **16**

7 Ductal Carcinoma In Situ (DCIS) in Sclerosing Adenosis vs Infiltrating Ductal Carcinoma **18**

8 Lobular Carcinoma In Situ (LCIS) in Sclerosing Adenosis vs Infiltrating Lobular Carcinoma **20**

9 Atypical Ductal Hyperplasia (ADH) and Ductal Carcinoma In Situ (DCIS) in Sclerosing Adenosis vs Atypical Lobular Hyperplasia (ALH) and Lobular Carcinoma In Situ (LCIS) in Sclerosing Adenosis **22**

SECTION 2: DUCTAL AND LOBULAR PROLIFERATIONS

10 Usual Hyperplasia vs ADH **26**

11 Usual Hyperplasia and ADH vs Low-Grade DCIS **30**

12 Low-Grade DCIS vs Intermediate and High-Grade DCIS **36**

13 Cribriform DCIS vs Infiltrating Cribriform Carcinoma **40**

14 Apocrine Hyperplasia and Atypical Apocrine Hyperplasia vs Apocrine DCIS **42**

15 Usual Lobular Hyperplasia and ALH vs LCIS **46**

16 Lobular Extension of DCIS vs Ductal Extension of LCIS **48**

17 Collagenous Spherulosis vs Cribriform DCIS and Adenoid Cystic Carcinoma **52**

SECTION 3: RADIAL SCARS, RADIAL SCLEROSING LESIONS, AND COMPLEX SCLEROSING LESIONS

18 Radial Sclerosing Lesions vs Infiltrating Carcinoma **55**

19 DCIS and ADH within Radial Sclerosing Lesions vs Usual Radial Scars and Infiltrating Carcinoma **58**

20 LCIS and ALH in Radial Sclerosing Lesions vs Infiltrating Carcinoma **62**

21 Postbiopsy and Traumatic Alterations in In Situ Carcinoma vs Infiltrating Carcinoma **64**

SECTION 4: PAPILLARY LESIONS

22 Papilloma vs Noninfiltrating Papillary Carcinoma (papillary DCIS) **69**

23 Papilloma with Sclerotic Alterations vs Infiltrating Ductal Carcinoma Associated with Papilloma **74**

24 Papilloma with Metaplastic Alterations vs Carcinoma **76**

25 Atypical Hyperplasia in Papilloma (Atypical Papilloma) vs DCIS Arising in Papilloma **80**

26 Infiltrating Papillary Carcinoma vs Non–infiltrating Papillary Carcinoma with Pseudoinfiltration **81**

SECTION 5: SPECIAL TYPES OF INFILTRATING CARCINOMA

27 Tubular Carcinoma vs Other Types of Infiltrating Ductal Carcinoma **84**

28 Infiltrating Cribriform Carcinoma vs DCIS of the Cribriform Type vs Adenoid Cystic Carcinoma and Other Types of Infiltrating Carcinoma **88**

29 Medullary Carcinoma vs Atypical Medullary Carcinoma vs Malignant Lymphoma **94**

30 Metaplastic Carcinoma vs Stromal Proliferations and Phyllodes Tumor **98**

31 Mucinous (Colloid) Carcinoma vs Mucocele-Like Lesions vs Cystic Hypersecretory Carcinoma vs Juvenile Papillomatosis **102**

32 Infiltrating Lobular Carcinoma of the Classical Type vs Other Patterns of Infiltrating Lobular Carcinoma **108**

SECTION 6: DISORDERS OF THE NIPPLE

33 Nipple Duct Adenoma (Florid Papillomatosis of the Nipple) vs Well-Differentiated Carcinoma vs Syringomatous Adenoma **114**

34 Paget Disease of the Nipple vs Cutaneous Tumors **120**

SECTION 7: BIPHASIC AND MESENCHYMAL PROLIFERATIONS

35 Fibroadenoma vs Low-Grade Phyllodes Tumor **128**

36 Juvenile Fibroadenoma vs Fibroadenoma of the Adult Type vs Low-Grade Phyllodes Tumor **136**

37 Fibroadenoma with Superimposed Sclerosing Adenosis vs Fibroadenoma with Infiltrating Carcinoma **138**

38 Low-Grade (Benign) Phyllodes Tumor vs High-Grade (Malignant) Phyllodes Tumor **140**

39 High-Grade Phyllodes Tumor with Sarcomatous Overgrowth vs Pure Sarcoma **142**

40 Periductal Stromal Sarcoma vs Phyllodes Tumor vs Pure Sarcoma **144**

41 Carcinosarcoma vs Metaplastic Carcinoma vs Pure Sarcoma **146**

42 Pseudoangiomatous Hyperplasia of Mammary Stroma vs Angiosarcoma **148**

43 Benign Vascular Proliferations vs Angiosarcoma **150**

44 Poorly Differentiated Angiosarcoma vs Other Malignant Spindle Cell Tumors **153**

45 Fibromatosis vs Fibrosarcoma vs Metaplastic Carcinoma **154**

46 Granular Cell Tumor vs Histiocytoid Carcinoma **156**

47 Fat Necrosis vs Histiocytoid Carcinoma vs Lipid-Rich Carcinoma **158**

SECTION 8: LESIONS INVOLVING AXILLARY LYMPH NODES

48 Capsular Nevus Cell Aggregates and Nodal Glandular Inclusions vs Metastatic Tumors **162**

49 Metastatic Lobular Carcinoma vs Sinus Histiocytosis **164**

50 Metastatic Lobular Carcinoma vs Malignant Lymphoma **165**

SECTION 9: SPECIMEN RADIOGRAPHS: WHAT TO LOOK FOR

51 Densities with Smooth Borders vs Densities with Spiculation or Distortion **168**

52 Highly Suspicious Calcifications vs Calcifications of Intermediate Concern **170**

SECTION 10: BIBLIOGRAPHY AND INDEX

Bibliography **177**

Index **183**

Section 1   ADENOSIS

GENERAL CONSIDERATIONS

Adenosis is a general term used to describe various nonneoplastic histologic alterations of the glandular elements of the mammary tissue, usually associated with expansion of the terminal ductal-lobular units. This expansion is a result of an increase in the number of ductules, as well as elongation of the ductules.

Several histologic variants of adenosis are recognized, only two of which have diagnostic usefulness: *sclerosing adenosis* (SA) and *microglandular adenosis* (MA). These are reasonably distinct entities with clinical correlates. SA is very common, whereas MA is rather rare. Other variants include so-called blunt duct adenosis, tubular adenosis, and secretory adenosis. Apocrine metaplasia with or without atypia is not uncommon in SA (*apocrine adenosis*), and some cases of this type have also been referred to as adenomyoepithelial adenosis by some authors. Both the usual and atypical forms of epithelial hyperplasia may develop in SA, as may lobular carcinoma in situ (LCIS) and ductal carcinoma in situ (DCIS). These secondary alterations may be confined to the area of SA or may extend into the lesion from the neighboring foci.

Different forms of adenosis, with or without superimposed metaplastic and proliferative alterations, may cause various differential diagnostic problems. These problems are discussed in the following chapters.

CLINICAL

Adenosis is usually seen in association with other fibrocystic alterations and generally affects women in the childbearing and perimenopausal years. Although it is usually a microscopic finding in the setting of fibrocystic changes, adenosis may also present as a mass lesion, which results from the coalescence of many adjacent lobules showing this alteration. This latter form of adenosis is variably referred to as *nodular adenosis*, *adenosis tumor*, *tumoral adenosis*, or *aggregate adenosis*. These mass lesions may be clinically palpable and may at times mimic carcinoma. However, although firm, they are characteristically mobile and rubbery masses and lack the clinical retraction signs. Regression of adenosis with menopause has been noted.

The relative risk of infiltrating breast carcinoma in patients with SA is approximately 1.7. Whether CIS in areas of SA is more frequently found in lesions presenting as a palpable mass (nodular adenosis) is not known. However, one-fifth to one-third of the cases of CIS reported as presenting in SA have involved palpable adenosis tumors. SA has also been shown to be associated with atypical lobular hyperplasia (ALH) three times more often than with other forms of fibrocystic disease. The clinical significance of atypical apocrine metaplasia in SA has not been clearly established, but follow-up of these patients is advised. On rare occasions, carcinomas have been reported in association with or arising in MA. Therefore, if MA shows atypical features, these patients should also be closely followed after surgical excision of the lesion.

IMAGING

All histologic patterns of adenosis may be associated with numerous small, punctuate microcalcifications on mammography that result from precipitated calcium salts within ductules of the expanded lobular units. SA has variable mammographic appearances. Diffuse or focally clustered microcalcifications of the lobular type are the most commonly reported findings. Rarely, a circumscribed or ill-defined mass with focal asymmetry may be present, which may or may not contain microcalcifications.

GROSS

Morphologically, the appearance of adenosis varies from microscopic alterations which are not grossly visible (most common form) to tumor-like nodular masses. The nodular forms of adenosis present as firm nodules that are fairly well demarcated from the surrounding breast tissue. The cut surfaces appear pink to light brown and bulging. These masses vary in size from a few millimeters to 2.5 cm. The appearance of some of these mass lesions may mimic carcinoma on gross examination. Their contours, however, although irregular, are often smooth and finely nodular, as opposed to the irregular, infiltrating, stellate periphery that is seen in the ordinary infiltrating carcinomas. The lesions are firm and rubbery but not hard or gritty in consistency, as they are in most infiltrating carcinomas with stromal fibrosis. In addition, they do not grossly resemble the circumscribed carcinoma variants such as medullary carcinoma and colloid carcinoma.

1. Sclerosing Adenosis vs Tubular Carcinoma

Sclerosing adenosis (SA) is a lobulocentric lesion characterized by enlargement of the terminal ductal-lobular units, with organoid proliferation and elongation of the ductules (Figs. 1.1–1.3). The lobulocentricity of SA can be easily appreciated when an early lesion is compared with a normal lobule (Figs. 1.2, 1.4). In this form of adenosis the proliferating ductular structures are enveloped and distorted by fibrosis, which produces irregular clusters and strands of epithelial nests within the altered fibrous stroma (Figs. 1.1–1.3). The stroma in SA is usually sparse but shows increased cellularity and fibrous alterations. When the epithelial proliferation is exuberant and fibrosis is minimal, the lesion may be referred to as *florid adenosis*. The two-cell population, for the most part, is retained. Myoepithelial cells may become spindled, clear or hyperplastic, and frequently rather prominent (Figs. 1.5, 1.6). Scattered and clustered, round intraluminal microcalcifications are fairly common. SA may focally extend into or push toward the surrounding adipose tissue, as may the normal lobules (Fig. 1.3).

Proliferating and distorted ductular units of *SA* may superficially mimic infiltrating ductal carcinoma, specifically the tubular type. The key to the differential diagnosis is the low-power examination. The lobulated, organoid arrangement of the ductules and rounded nodular periphery are characteristic of SA (Figs. 1.1, 1.2). Ductules are usually arranged in a parallel (streaming) fashion, with central attenuation in size and partial obliteration of the lumina. As a result, the central portion of the lesion appears most cellular on low-power examination (Figs. 1.1–1.3). At higher magnification, ductular structures with a distinct but centrally attenuated lumen and a surrounding basement membrane are easily identified (Figs. 1.5, 1.6). The attenu-

ated ductules are lined by both epithelial and myoepithelial cells, but the two-cell population may be difficult to distinguish in some of the ductules (Fig. 1.5).

In contrast, *tubular carcinoma (TC)* shows an irregular periphery (Figs. 1.7, 1.8). The ducts of TC are haphazardly distributed and slightly variable but fairly uniform in size, and maintain a well-differentiated tubular appearance with angulated shapes and open lumina throughout (Figs. 1.7–1.9). The central portion of the lesion may show dense fibrosis and elastosis, but the stroma is usually reactive-appearing and fibroblastic (Fig. 1.9). In TC the neoplastic ducts are lined by a single type of epithelial cell with fairly uniform nuclei and inconspicuous nucleoli (Figs. 1.8, 1.9). Occasional luminal bridges and cribriform patterns may be present (Figs. 1.7, 1.9). Mitotic figures and pleomorphism are not prominent. The myoepithelial cells and basal lamina are absent (Fig. 1.9).

Although *SA* may push toward or extend into the adipose tissue, the lobular pattern with a nodular, circumscribed periphery is characteristically maintained (Figs. 1.1, 1.2). *TC*, in contrast, is characterized by neoplastic ducts which infiltrate the adjacent stroma and adipose tissue (Figs. 1.7, 1.8).

A periodic acid–Schiff (PAS) stain demonstrates the presence of basement membrane around the ductules in *SA.* In addition, immunostains for smooth muscle actin demonstrate the presence of myoepithelial cells (Fig. 1.10A). Both techniques help to further distinguish *SA* from *TC*, the glands of which lack both basal lamina and myoepithelium (Fig. 1.10B).

The two-cell composition of adenosis can be demonstrated in fine needle aspiration (FNA) preparations (Fig. 1.11). This contrasts with the uniform, monomorphic cell population characteristic of *TC* (Fig. 1.12).

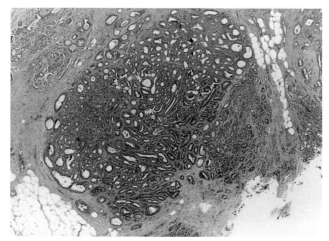

Figure 1.1. Sclerosing adenosis.

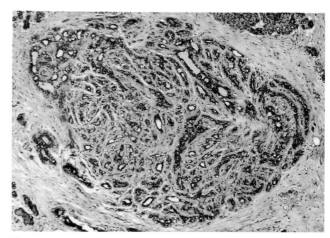

Figure 1.2. Sclerosing adenosis.

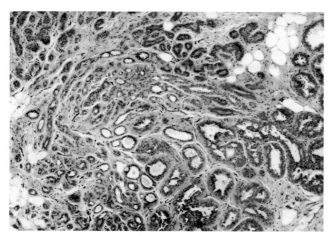

Figure 1.3. Sclerosing adenosis.

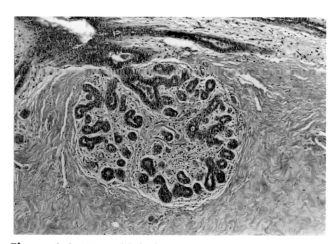

Figure 1.4. Normal lobule.

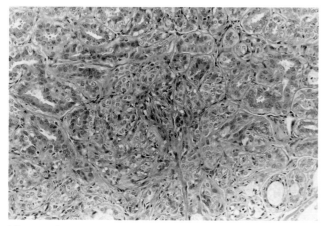

Figure 1.5. Sclerosing adenosis.

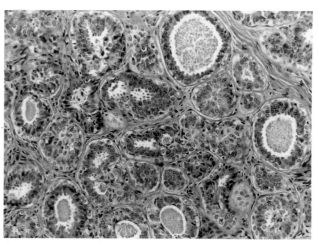

Figure 1.6. Sclerosing adenosis.

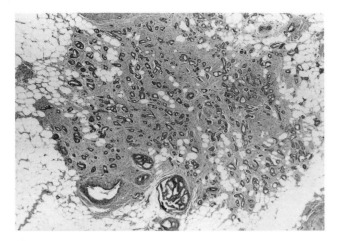

Figure 1.7. Tubular carcinoma.

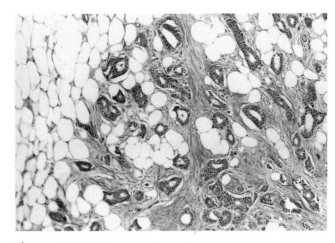

Figure 1.8. Tubular carcinoma.

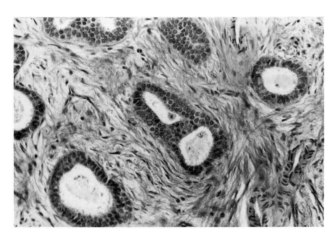

Figure 1.9. Tubular carcinoma.

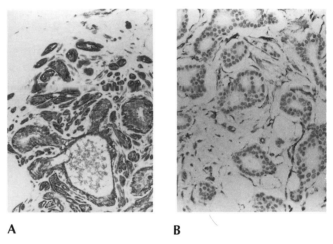

A   B

Figure 1.10A. Sclerosing adenosis. Actin immunoperoxidase. **B.** Tubular carcinoma. Actin immunoperoxidase.

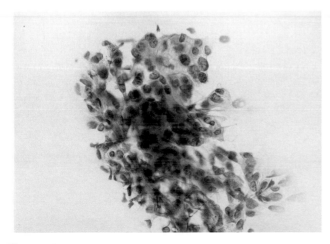

Figure 1.11. Adenosis. FNA.

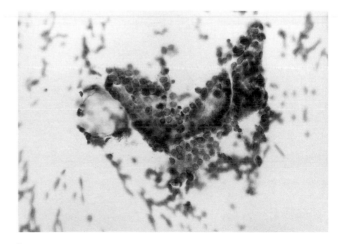

Figure 1.12. Tubular carcinoma. FNA.

2. Perineural Space Extension in Sclerosing Adenosis vs Perineural Invasion by Infiltrating Carcinoma

In *SA*, proliferating, distorted ductular structures may *surround the nerves or extend into the perineural space* (Figs. 2.1, 2.2) and, rarely may even be present within the substance of the nerve. These infrequent findings may mimic *perineural space invasion or neural invasion* occurring with *infiltrating ductal carcinoma* (Figs. 2.3–2.6). However, once the previously discussed benign histologic and cytologic features of SA and its individual glands are recognized in the perineural area and the surrounding tissue, the issue is no longer problematic (Figs. 2.1, 2.2).

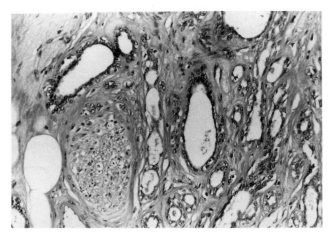

Figure 2.1. Perineural extension in sclerosing adenosis.

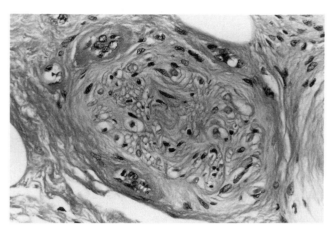

Figure 2.2. Perineural extension in sclerosing adenosis.

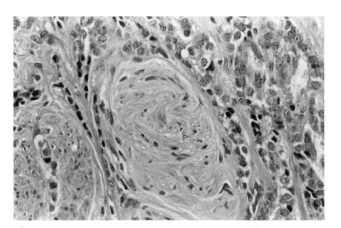

Figure 2.3. Perineural invasion in infiltrating carcinoma.

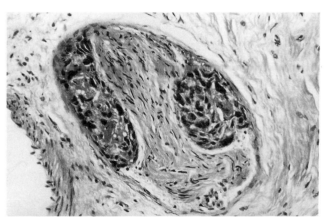

Figure 2.4. Perineural invasion in infiltrating carcinoma.

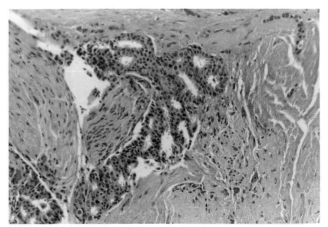

Figure 2.5. Perineural invasion in infiltrating carcinoma.

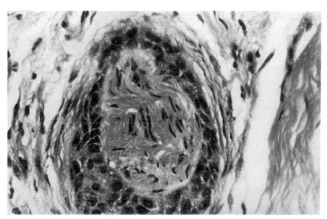

Figure 2.6. Perineural invasion in infiltrating carcinoma.

3. Nonneoplastic Apocrine Alterations in Sclerosing Adenosis vs Apocrine Carcinoma

Apocrine alterations comprise some of the more difficult differential diagnostic problems in breast pathology. When they involve the proliferating and distorted ductular units of *SA*, the problems are compounded. These apocrine alterations, which apply to ductal lesions in general, have been clearly outlined and described by Tavassoli and Norris (1994).

Apocrine metaplasia may occur in SA. These metaplastic cells are often large and irregularly arranged, and show abundant eosinophilic, granular to focally clear cytoplasm and enlarged, round, vesicular or oval nuclei, commonly with prominent round nucleoli (Fig. 3.1). The above-mentioned cytologic changes of apocrine metaplasia in *SA* (apocrine adenosis) are not considered atypical. However, if the nuclei display at least a threefold variation in size and there is no proliferation of cells, the lesions qualify as atypical apocrine metaplasia, which generally involves *SA*. If, in addition, the apocrine cell population showing variable degrees of atypia also undergoes hyperplastic changes, such as tufting, papillary formations and stratification, or bridges, arcades and a cribriform arrangement, then the possibilities of atypical apocrine hyperplasia and noncomedo types (low and intermediate grades) of apocrine DCIS involving *SA* must be considered (Figs. 3.2–3.5). The comedo (necrotic) type (high grade) of apocrine DCIS in adenosis is usually not difficult to recognize because of the markedly atypical nature of the apocrine cells and the presence of central necrosis. On the other hand, because of the distorted nature of the ductules in *SA*, the distinction between atypical apocrine hyperplasia and apocrine DCIS of the lower-grade noncomedo type may only be possible after examination of the adjacent parenchyma and identification there of the diagnostic features of these lesions. These differential diagnostic criteria, which apply to apocrine ductal proliferations in general, will be discussed in more detail in Section 2.

When the above–described metaplastic, hyperplastic, and neoplastic apocrine alterations involve the markedly distorted ductular units of *SA*, then the lesions may resemble *infiltrating apocrine carcinoma* (Figs 3.6–3.8). In differentiating these secondary apocrine changes in *SA* from infiltrating apocrine carcinoma, the general criteria used to distinguish atypical, hyperplastic, and in situ neoplastic alterations of the nonapocrine type involving SA from infiltrating carcinoma without apocrine features are used. The first step is low-power examination of the lesion and the surrounding breast tissue. Recognition of the lobulocentricity of SA, and the absence of in situ or invasive apocrine carcinoma within SA and in the surrounding breast tissue, indicate that these changes represent usual or atypical apocrine metaplasia in *SA* (apocrine adenosis) (Figs. 3.7, 3.8). However, if the histologic patterns or cytologic features of atypical apocrine hyperplasia or apocrine DCIS are recognized within SA or in the adjacent breast parenchyma, and if the distorted ductular structures of SA are involved by these cells, distinction from infiltrating apocrine carcinoma may be even more difficult (Figs. 3.6, 3.9, 3.10). Findings helpful in this distinction are (1) the presence of basement membrane around the proliferating ductules, which contain atypical cells in SA, and (2) the focal presence of residual myoepithelial cells within these ductules (Figs. 3.8–3.10). Both of these features are absent in infiltrating apocrine carcinoma (Figs. 3.11, 3.12). When there is doubt, however, a PAS stain and immunostains for actin may be performed, and these may provide further documentation.

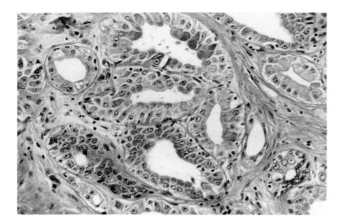

Figure 3.1. Apocrine metaplasia in adenosis.

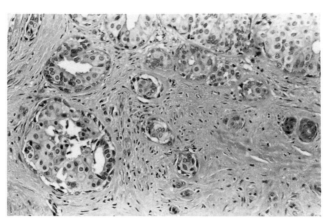

Figure 3.2. Atypical apocrine hyperplasia in sclerosing adenosis.

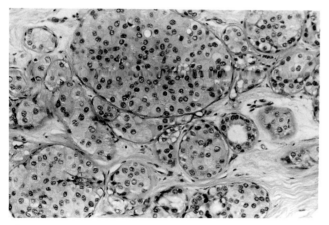

Figure 3.3. Apocrine ductal carcinoma in situ, low-grade, in adenosis.

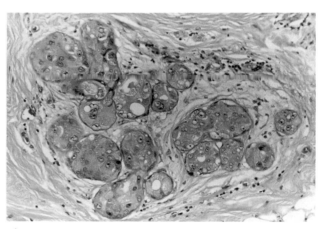

Figure 3.4. Apocrine ductal carcinoma in situ in adenosis.

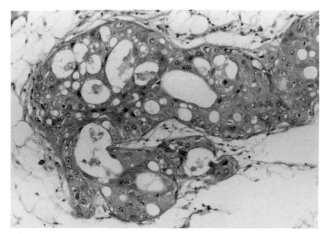

Figure 3.5. Apocrine ductal carcinoma in situ extending into adenosis.

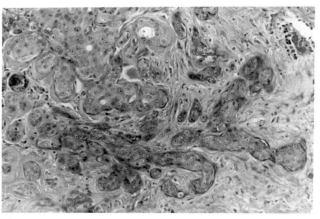

Figure 3.6. Apocrine ductal carcinoma in situ extending into sclerosing adenosis.

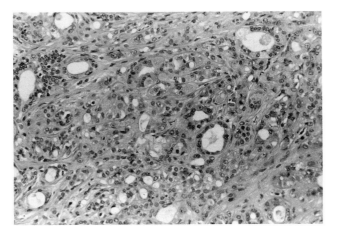

Figure 3.7. Apocrine metaplasia in sclerosing adenosis.

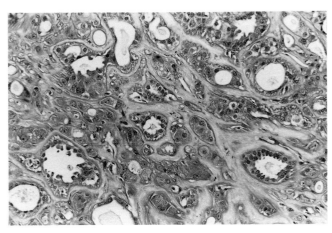

Figure 3.8. Atypical apocrine metaplasia in sclerosing adenosis.

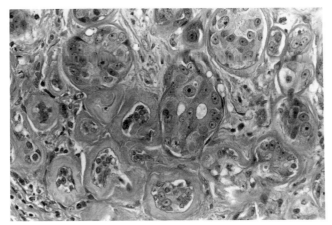

Figure 3.9. Apocrine ductal carcinoma in situ in sclerosing adenosis.

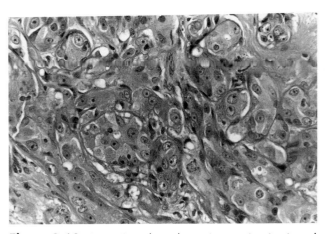

Figure 3.10. Apocrine ductal carcinoma in situ in sclerosing adenosis.

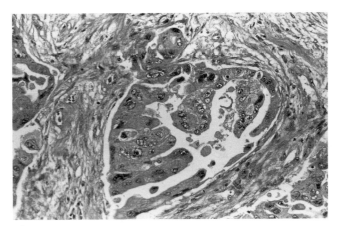

Figure 3.11. Infiltrating apocrine carcinoma.

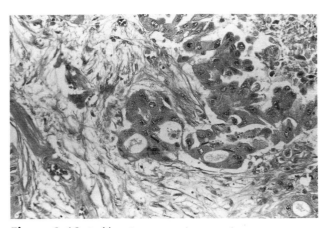

Figure 3.12. Infiltrating apocrine carcinoma.

4. Sclerosing Adenosis with Marked Ductular Attenuation vs Infiltrating Lobular Carcinoma

Attenuated ductular structures in SA may, on rare occasions, resemble foci of *infiltrating lobular carcinoma* (Figs. 4.1, 4.2). A nodular, lobulocentric configuration of SA on low-power examination is the key to this differential diagnosis (Fig. 4.3). In addition, the cells in question in SA are often spindled (myoepithelial cells) and lack the cytologic features of LCIS cells (Figs. 4.1, 4.5). In *infiltrating lobular carcinoma*, on the other hand, lobulocentricity is absent but multiple isolated microscopic foci may be present (Fig. 4.4). The neoplastic cells are round and arranged in rigid linear arrays, and a variable population may have intracytoplasmic lumina (Figs. 4.2, 4.6).

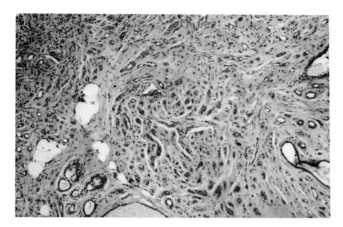

Figure 4.1. Sclerosing adenosis with attenuated ductules.

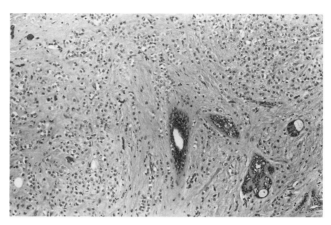

Figure 4.2. Infiltrating lobular carcinoma.

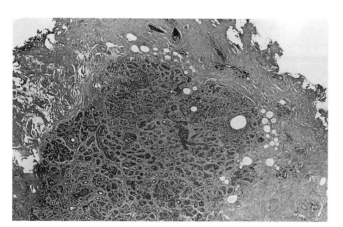

Figure 4.3. Sclerosing adenosis.

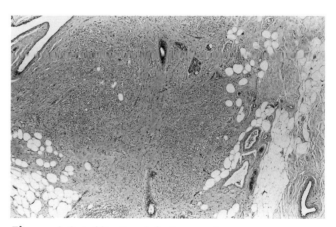

Figure 4.4. Infiltrating lobular carcinoma.

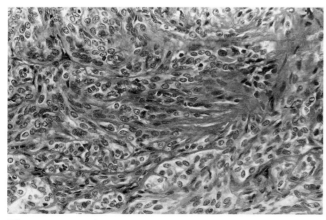

Figure 4.5. Sclerosing adenosis.

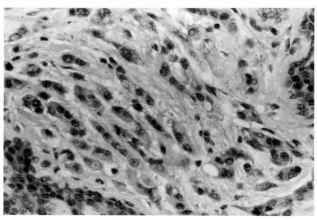

Figure 4.6. Infiltrating lobular carcinoma.

5. Microglandular Adenosis vs Tubular Carcinoma

Microglandular adenosis (MA) is a rare form of adenosis. It is not a lobulocentric lesion and is characterized by proliferation of small, round, fairly uniform glandular structures with no organoid orientation. The glands are distributed haphazardly within the stroma and may extend into the fat (Figs. 5.1–5.3). In some areas they appear "naked" in the adipose tissue or fibrous breast stroma (Figs. 5.1–5.3). The glands are round to oval in shape and usually exhibit open lumina, although the lumina of the smaller glands may be narrow or closed (Figs. 5.1–5.3). They frequently contain PAS-positive and sometimes mucicarmine- and alcian blue–positive secretory material (Figs. 5.2, 5.3). Scattered foci of luminal calcification may also be present. The glands are lined by a single layer of cuboidal epithelial cells, with clear to eosinophilic cytoplasm and round to oval, bland nuclei (Fig. 5.3). The myoepithelial cell layer is usually absent, but some authors have demonstrated the presence of rare myoepithelial cells by immunohistochemical stains. However, these lesions probably represent examples of so-called secretory adenosis (which characteristically has a myoepithelial layer) rather than MA. The stroma in MA may be dense and collagenized or loose and hypocellular (Figs. 5.1, 5.2).

Since the ductular units of *MA* are not arranged in an organoid pattern and extend haphazardly through the stroma and adipose tissue, without a recognizable myoepithelial layer this lesion may be confused with *TC*. In distinguishing these two lesions, it is important to recognize that the glands of *MA* have a small, round, uniform appearance. The lining epithelial cells are usually bland, may have cytoplasmic vacuolization, and show truncated luminal margins. Eosinophilic luminal secretions are often prominent (Figs. 5.1–5.3).

In contrast, the glands of *TC* are slightly irregular, angulated or oval in shape, and lack luminal secretions. Apical snouts are characteristically present (Figs. 5.4, 5.5). In addition, luminal bridges may be seen focally in TC (Fig. 5.5), as well as an associated low-grade DCIS. Neither of these features should be seen in uncomplicated MA. Lastly, in *MA* the stroma is often relatively acellular and hyalinized (Figs. 5.1, 5.2), whereas in *TC* it may show fibrosis and elastosis but may often be reactive-appearing and fibroblastic (Figs. 5.4, 5.5).

Immunohistochemically, the glands of *MA* are epithelial membrane antigen (EMA) negative and show distinct basal lamina, as demonstrated by PAS stain. In *TC*, on the other hand, basal lamina is usually absent, as demonstrated by PAS stain, and EMA antibody strongly stains the glycocalyx of the neoplastic glands. Generally, no myoepithelial cells can be demonstrated by actin immunostains in either lesion (Figs. 5.6A, 5.6B).

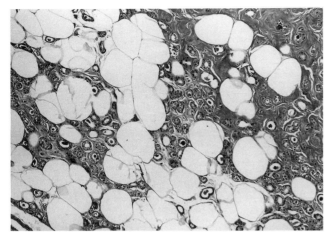

Figure 5.1. Microglandular adenosis.

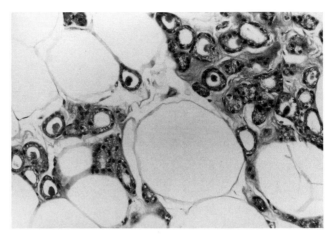

Figure 5.2. Microglandular adenosis.

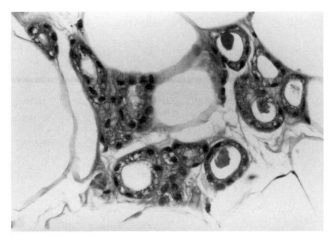

Figure 5.3. Microglandular adenosis.

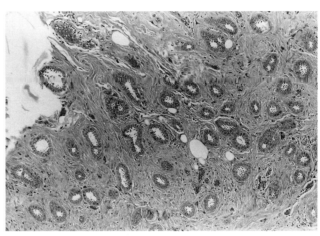

Figure 5.4. Tubular carcinoma.

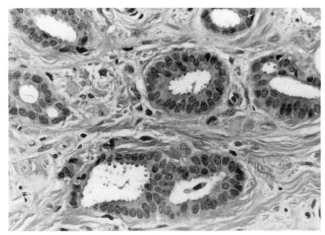

Figure 5.5. Tubular carcinoma.

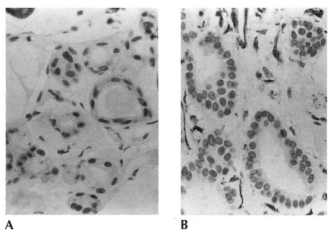

A   B

Figure 5.6A. Microglandular adenosis. Actin immunoperoxidase. **B.** Tubular carcinoma. Actin immunoperoxidase.

6. Sclerosing Adenosis vs Radial Scars and Complex Sclerosing Lesions (Radial Sclerosing Lesions)

Radial scars and complex sclerosing lesions may at times resemble *SA*. Once again, the low-power examination is the key in this differential diagnosis. *SA* has a lobulated outline (Figs. 6.1, 6.2), and the central portion of the lesion is hypercellular due to the presence of crowded, compressed ductules (Figs. 6.1, 6.3A). Elastosis is unusual. Peripherally, the lobulocentric pattern, with smooth contours and usually open ductules, is preserved (Figs. 6.1, 6.2, 6.3B). Two-cell-layer lining epithelium is maintained (Fig. 6.3B).

Radial scars, on the other hand, have a stellate periphery (Fig. 6.4). The central area is poorly cellular and shows fibrosis and elastosis, with entrapment of the ductules (Figs. 6.4–6.6). The ductules surrounding this area are arranged in a radial fashion (Figs. 6.4, 6.5). They are lined by epithelial and myoepithelial cells and may show epithelial proliferation of varying degrees and patterns (Figs. 6.4–6.6A, B). These lesions and their accompanying differential diagnostic problems will be discussed in detail in Section 3.

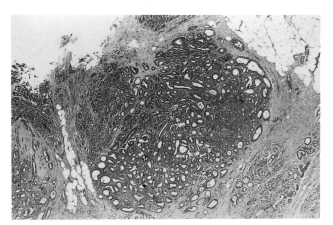

Figure 6.1. Sclerosing adenosis.

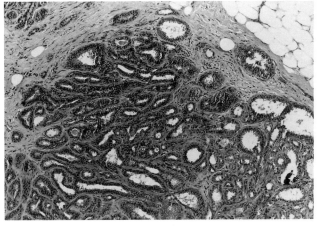

Figure 6.2. Sclerosing adenosis.

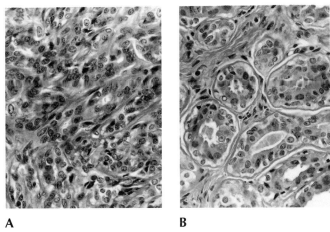

A   B

Figure 6.3A. Sclerosing adenosis, central portion.
B. Sclerosing adenosis, peripheral portion.

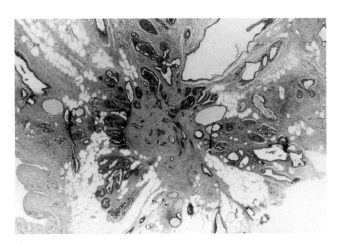

Figure 6.4. Radial scar.

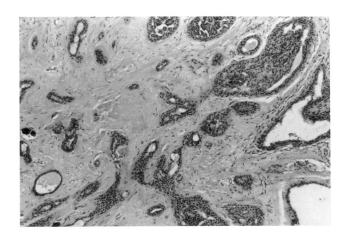

Figure 6.5. Radial scar.

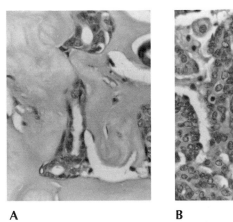

A   B

Figure 6.6A. Radial scar, central portion. **B.** Radial scar, peripheral portion.

7. Ductal Carcinoma In Situ (DCIS) in Sclerosing Adenosis vs Infiltrating Ductal Carcinoma

DCIS extending into or developing within the proliferating and deformed units of *SA* may mimic *infiltrating ductal carcinoma* and may present difficulties in diagnosis (Figs. 7.1, 7.2). Under low-power examination, recognition of the benign organoid nature of background SA is the initial step in making the correct diagnosis (Fig. 7.1). The classic histologic patterns and cytologic features of DCIS associated with SA are usually not difficult to identify (Figs. 7.3, 7.4). However, due to the distorted nature of the ductules in SA, the distinction between ADH and DCIS involving SA may not be possible without examination of the adjacent breast parenchyma and identification there of the diagnostic features.

To distinguish the distorted glandular structures of SA involved by DCIS cells from the infiltrating glands of infiltrating ductal carcinoma, the following additional features are helpful: (1) a well-defined basement membrane around the distorted, proliferating ductules containing neoplastic cells within the SA and (2) focal residual myoepithelial cells within these ductules (Figs. 7.1, 7.2). Both of these features are absent in infiltrating ductal carcinoma (Figs. 7.5, 7.6).

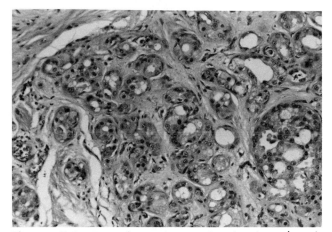

Figure 7.1. Ductal carcinoma in situ in sclerosing adenosis.

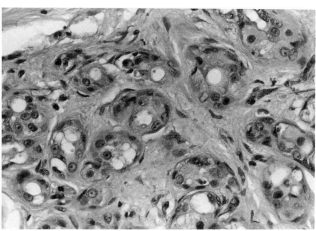

Figure 7.2. Ductal carcinoma in situ in sclerosing adenosis.

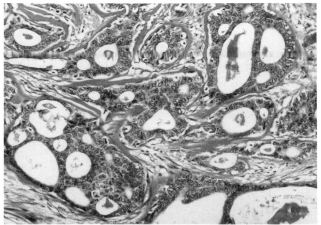

Figure 7.3. Ductal carcinoma in situ extending into adenosis.

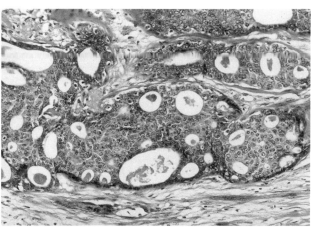

Figure 7.4. Ductal carcinoma in situ extending into adenosis.

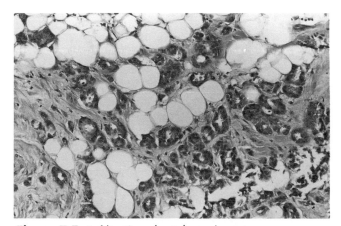

Figure 7.5. Infiltrating ductal carcinoma.

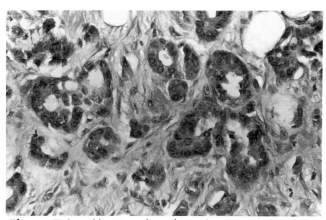

Figure 7.6. Infiltrating ductal carcinoma.

8. Lobular Carcinoma In Situ (LCIS) in Sclerosing Adenosis vs Infiltrating Lobular Carcinoma

LCIS which colonizes or arises within areas of *SA* may also resemble infiltrating lobular carcinoma (Figs. 8.1–8.4). As in DCIS within SA, the low-power microscopic examination is the key. Once the lobulated, organoid appearance of background SA is recognized and the appropriate cytologic features of LCIS are observed within the ductular units of the lesion, and if the fully developed lesions of LCIS are present in areas outside of the adenosis, the diagnosis of LCIS in SA is not difficult (Figs. 8.2–8.4). The demonstration of intracytoplasmic mucin droplets may also be helpful in distinguishing LCIS in adenosis from florid forms of adenosis (Fig. 8.4).

However, when the centrally compressed and markedly attenuated units of SA are involved with LCIS cells, the appearance may mimic that of *infiltrating lobular carcinoma* (Fig. 8.5). The presence of an intact basement membrane surrounding the distorted ductular units filled with neoplastic cells and the persistence of residual myoepithelial cells are helpful in determining that these areas do not represent invasive neoplasm (Figs. 8.1–8.3, 8.5). Both of these findings (which may at times require special stains for definite documentation) are absent in infiltrating lobular carcinoma (Fig. 8.6). Although on rare occasions some of the neoplastic cells may appear to be isolated in the stroma of SA, as long as they remain confined to the framework and configuration of SA the lesion is considered noninvasive.

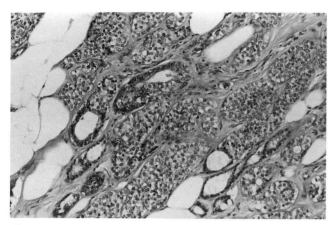

Figure 8.1. Lobular carcinoma in situ in adenosis.

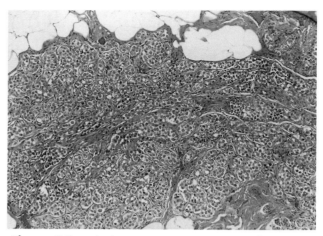

Figure 8.2. Lobular carcinoma in situ in adenosis.

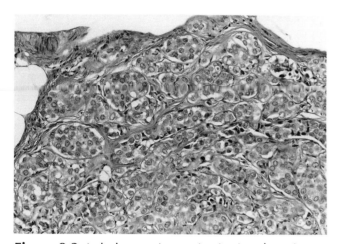

Figure 8.3. Lobular carcinoma in situ in adenosis.

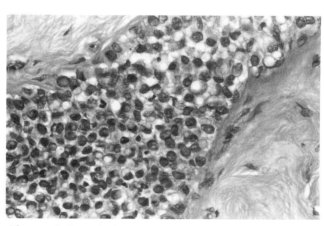

Figure 8.4. Lobular carcinoma in situ, cellular detail.

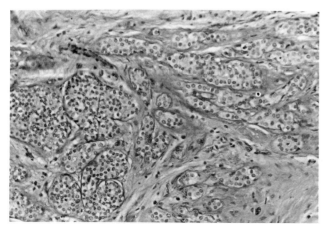

Figure 8.5. Lobular carcinoma in situ in sclerosing adenosis.

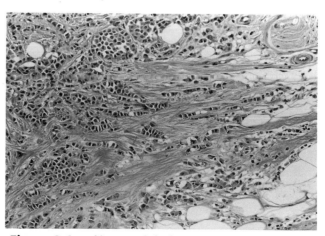

Figure 8.6. Infiltrating lobular carcinoma.

9. Atypical Ductal Hyperplasia (ADH) and Ductal Carcinoma In Situ (DCIS) in Sclerosing Adenosis vs Atypical Lobular Hyperplasia (ALH) and Lobular Carcinoma In Situ (LCIS) in Sclerosing Adenosis

Once the low-power pattern of background SA is recognized, the standard criteria used to differentiate *ADH* from *DCIS* are applied to diagnose the superimposed ductal lesion. These criteria will be defined and discussed in detail in Section 2. However, in many cases, it is not possible to distinguish adenosis colonized by *ADH* from that associated with *DCIS* due to the narrow, compressed nature of the ductules in SA. In such cases, it is necessary to recognize the fully developed lesions of ADH or DCIS in the adjacent tissue away from the distorted ductules of SA for a definitive diagnosis.

Similarly, when the ductules of SA contain the cells characteristic of lobular neoplasia and when the spaces appear to be expanded or filled, *ALH* can be diagnosed. However, for the diagnosis of *LCIS in SA*, all of the material, including the areas free of distortion by the adenosis, should be carefully examined for characteristic features of LCIS. These features will also be defined and discussed in detail in Section 2.

In addition, DCIS colonizing or arising in SA must be distinguished from LCIS within adenosis. The cells of DCIS involving the distorted, proliferating ductules of SA are generally more pleomorphic and larger than the cells of LCIS (Figs. 9.1–9.3). Cells of lobular neoplasia, on the other hand, are usually more uniform (Figs. 9.4–9.6). In some low-grade DCIS lesions, however, the cells may also be smaller and more uniform (Fig. 9.1). In this setting and in general, the presence of distinct cohesive cell borders and the formation of secondary lumina are the features that support the diagnosis of DCIS (Figs. 9.1, 9.3). In contrast, the presence of intracellular lumina containing mucin droplets favors lobular neoplasia (Fig. 9.6).

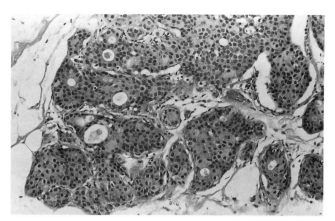

Figure 9.1. Ductal carcinoma in situ in adenosis, low grade.

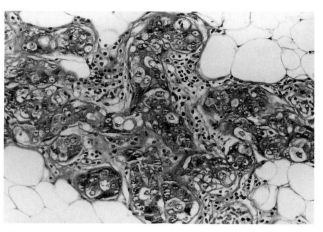

Figure 9.2. Ductal carcinoma in situ in adenosis.

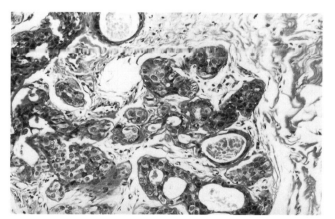

Figure 9.3. Ductal carcinoma in situ in adenosis.

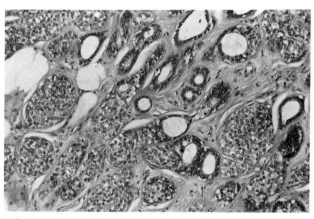

Figure 9.4. Lobular carcinoma in situ in adenosis.

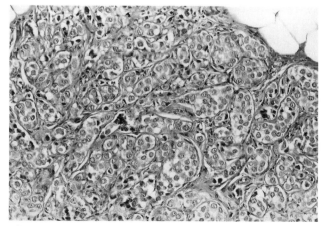

Figure 9.5. Lobular carcinoma in situ in adenosis.

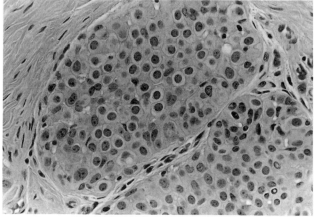

Figure 9.6. Lobular carcinoma in situ, cellular detail.

Section 2

DUCTAL AND LOBULAR PROLIFERATIONS

GENERAL CONSIDERATIONS

The term *ductal hyperplasia* designates the proliferation of epithelial and myoepithelial cells within ductal and lobular passages. Since this pattern of hyperplasia also involves both terminal ducts and smaller ductules (acini) of the lobule, there is an increasing tendency to use the terms *usual* or *ordinary hyperplasia* rather than *ductal hyperplasia*. In many instances the usual hyperplasic proliferations expand the smaller passages, so that lobules become filled and distended by the cells; as a result, these lobules resemble ducts histologically.

Other terms that have been used for these non-atypical hyperplastic proliferations include papillomatosis and epitheliosis. The term papillomatosis, however, has been used rather loosely in this context. The epithelial hyperplasias of the fenestrated type discussed in this section are not supported by fibrovascular stromal cores and should probably not be designated as papillomatosis (see also Section 4). Whichever term is selected by the pathologist, the true significance lies in distinguishing these lesions from atypical ductal and lobular hyperplasia and from ductal carcinoma in situ.

CLINICAL

Ductal (usual) *hyperplasia* is commonly seen in association with other fibrocystic alterations and more frequently affects women in the childbearing and perimenopausal years. Hyperplasia may at times be etiologically related to the formation of cysts in such conditions as juvenile papillomatosis (Swiss cheese disease). In that disorder, hyperplastic proliferations in terminal ducts are associated with cystic dilation of the adjacent lobules, apparently due to increased secretion of fluid or to the obstruction of terminal ducts.

Recent studies by Page and others have indicated that women with biopsies demonstrating usual hyperplasia of moderate to marked degree have a slightly increased relative risk (i.e., in the 1.5–2× range) of subsequently developing invasive mammary carcinoma. This compares to a 4–5× relative risk of developing carcinoma for the atypical lobular and ductal hyperplasias and a 9–10× relative risk of developing carcinoma for low-grade (noncomedo) intraductal carcinoma.

The probability of subsequent invasion by any particular instance of DCIS is not known. Studies indicate that high-grade DCIS lesions, such as most types of comedo carcinoma, are at greatest risk for recurrence and potentially aggressive behavior if they are not adequately excised. Low-grade DCIS lesions, on the other hand, are least likely to recur. Whether the majority of them would ultimately invade if left undiscovered is not known.

Micropapillary DCIS tends toward extensive local spread within the ductal passages. Free surgical margins may be more difficult to obtain with micropapillary DCIS than with other types of DCIS.

IMAGING

Moderate to florid hyperplastic proliferations may occasionally undergo sclerosis similar to that affecting papillary proliferations. Scarring within these lesions may produce irregular density, spiculation, or distortion, which can be detected on a mammogram.

In many cases, *usual* and *atypical hyperplasias* may be associated with clusters of calcifications similar to those seen in low-grade noncomedo types of DCIS. Small, rounded, benign-appearing calcifications characteristically occur in the more distal lobular units. Elongated ductal calcifications are less common but more suspicious, particularly in distended terminal ducts. Histologically, the calcifications associated with hyperplasia nearly always represent precipitation of secreted calcium salts. Significant necrosis is very uncommon in these lesions, and the linear and branching types of casting calcifications usually seen in high-grade comedo carcinoma do not occur.

Calcifications which develop within *DCIS* vary considerably in appearance, depending primarily on the presence or absence of central luminal necrosis. Many high-grade DCIS lesions demonstrate the comedo pattern of necrosis, in which calcifications develop within the necrotic debris and form a calcified "cast" of the duct lumen. The calcifications seen in these lesions on a mammogram characteristically have a linear and branching configuration, sometimes described as "casting calcifications" or as having a "dot-dash" appearance.

Calcifications which develop in lower-grade DCIS lesions, particularly the cribriform pattern of intraductal carcinoma, may have a more granular appearance and in most cases appear much less suspicious than those of high-grade DCIS. Many cases of low-grade intraductal carcinoma have none or few calcifications; the extent of these lesions may be difficult or impossible to document radiographically. LCIS and atypical lobular hyperplasia are usually not associated with calcifications.

GROSS

Hyperplastic and neoplastic lesions of ducts and lobules are generally not associated with grossly identifiable lesions unless there is periductal fibrosis, comedo necrosis, or scar formation. In many instances, attention is drawn to an area of hyperplasia because of nearby cyst formation; this is particularly true of the clustered pattern of cysts associated with juvenile papillomatosis. Large, florid, hyperplastic proliferations sometimes undergo radial scar formation, with the development of firm or spiculated masses. These proliferations may appear grossly suspicious for carcinoma. When comedo-type necrosis occurs in the higher-grade DCIS lesions, the yellow-white necrotic debris which protrudes from the cut surface of ducts is characteristic, but it cannot always be distinguished grossly from duct ectasia or small cysts containing inspissated material.

10. Usual Hyperplasia vs ADH

Usual hyperplasia of ductal and lobular spaces is an intraluminal proliferation of epithelial and myoepithelial cells. Since this is a dual-cell proliferation, the hyperplasia is not monotonous, but commonly appears as a gentle pleomorphic cellular proliferation which may seem to stream or swirl (Figs. 10.1, 10.2). Epithelial bridges in usual hyperplasia are typically delicate, not stiff (Fig. 10.3), and are composed of cells of varied appearance, at least one of which is often spindly (Fig. 10.4).

Another structural feature associated with moderate and florid degrees of usual hyperplasia is a tendency to form narrow secondary spaces within the lumen of the duct or lobule. These spaces often have a "collapsible" appearance, as if the weight of the cellular proliferation was compressing the spaces into narrow slits (Figs. 10.1, 10.4). Where large masses of cells are proliferating, they are commonly solid in the midportion of the space, with multiple narrow spaces in peripheral locations closer to the duct wall (Fig. 10.5). Occasionally some of the spaces in a lesion of usual hyperplasia may have a more worrisome, rounded appearance, but these rounded spaces are not generally distributed throughout the ductal space, nor are they entirely lined by uniform cells.

Cytologically, the cells of usual hyperplasia appear variable, characterized by differences in nuclear and cytoplasmic shape and by differences in the intensity of nuclear staining and cytoplasmic coloration (Fig. 10.6). Commonly, the primary cell type proliferating in usual hyperplasia appears to be similar to normal duct epithelial cells. The secondary cells resemble the myoepithelial cells normally seen beneath the epithelial cells in the duct wall (Fig. 10.4). In fact, it is sometimes helpful to identify the myoepithelial cell in its usual location, noting whether the nucleus is spindly or lymphocyte-like and then determining whether such a cell is participating in the luminal proliferation. Cytoplasmic alterations may also be helpful, particularly when the myoepithelial cytoplasm appears clear or vacuolated (Figs. 10.2, 10.6) or when features of apocrine metaplasia are present. Cell borders are usually ill defined in usual hyperplasia.

The cells in usual hyperplasia are not necessarily small. All cell types may appear enlarged; and this is not considered an indicator of atypia. Sometimes the myoepithelial cells are particularly enlarged, show proliferative alterations, and demonstrate abundant pale cytoplasm.

In general, the "spindly" cell shape and a swirling pattern are frequent features of usual hyperplasia. These features are particularly helpful in analyzing bridges and the round or punched-out-appearing spaces. If some of the cells appear to run along the bridge or around the lumen of a space in a spindly parallel fashion, this is a strong indicator of hyperplasia of the usual type (Fig. 10.6).

The term *atypical ductal hyperplasia (ADH)* is used to designate proliferations composed in part, but not entirely, of cell populations characteristically seen in low-grade noncomedo DCIS. The pathologist may identify characteristic features of both usual hyperplasia and noncomedo DCIS within the same space. Criteria for ADH have been well delineated by Page and others, and recent studies have confirmed the intermediate level of risk associated with these atypical lesions.

The development of an atypical cell population is recognized by two types of changes. (1) cytologic atypia, usually characterized by cellular uniformity and monomorphism, and (2) structural rigidity. When making a diagnosis of ADH, a portion of the membrane lined space must lack the atypical cellular changes, either by the persistence of a usual hyperplastic component such as spindly cells or by having portions of the wall lined by normal epithelia (Figs. 10.7–10.9).

Cytologic atypia in ADH is characterized by the presence of a population of low-grade cells demonstrating a nearly pure, uniform monomorphic population, with each cell appearing almost identical to the next and with little admixture of myoepithelial cells (Figs 10.7, 10.8). Cell borders are usually more distinct than those seen in usual hyperplasia, and the cells are more commonly hyperchromatic (Figs. 10.7, 10.8).

Structural atypia in ADH includes several patterns characteristic of DCIS, such as structural stiffness or rigidity (Fig. 10.7), a tendency toward crisp, punched-out spaces and Roman bridge formations (Figs. 10.8, 10.10), or formation of micropapillary excrescences (Fig. 10.9). A bridge formation in usual hyperplasia, for example, tends to taper, with some component of longitudinally oriented or spindly cells. By contrast, ADH is characterized by stiff, nontapering bars composed of uniform, evenly spaced cells (Fig. 10.7). A significant accumulation of uniform monomorphic cells, particularly in association with crisp spaces, may be interpreted as atypical hyperplasia (Figs. 10.11, 10.12).

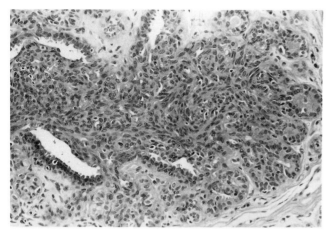

Figure 10.1. Usual hyperplasia.

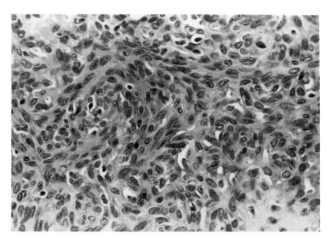

Figure 10.2. Usual hyperplasia.

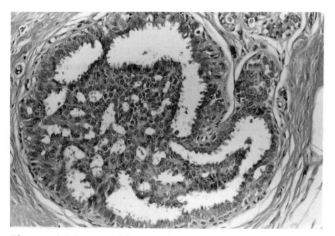

Figure 10.3. Usual hyperplasia.

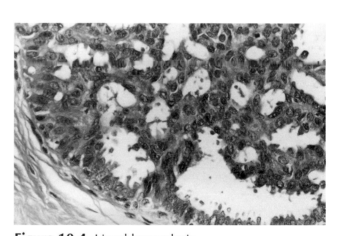

Figure 10.4. Usual hyperplasia.

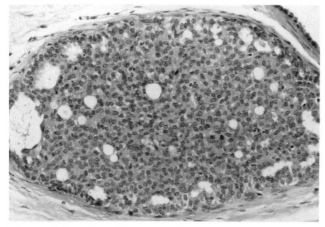

Figure 10.5. Usual hyperplasia.

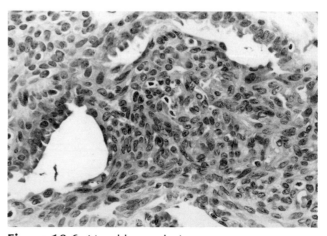

Figure 10.6. Usual hyperplasia.

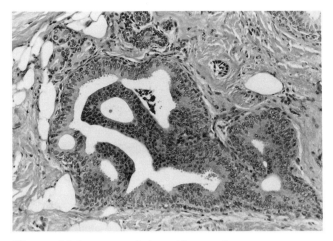

Figure 10.7. Atypical ductal hyperplasia.

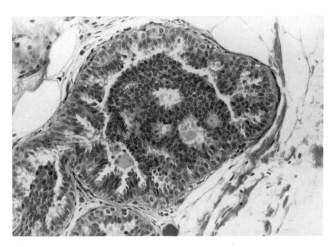

Figure 10.8. Atypical ductal hyperplasia.

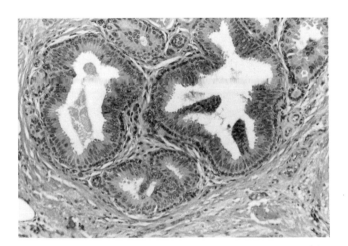

Figure 10.9. Atypical ductal hyperplasia.

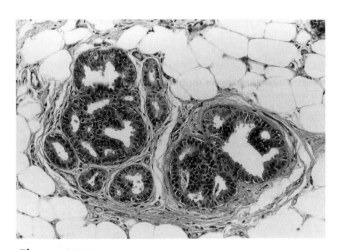

Figure 10.10. Atypical ductal hyperplasia.

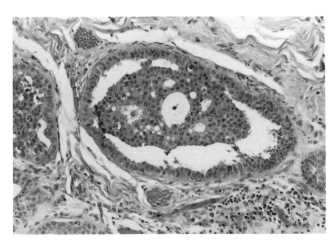

Figure 10.11. Atypical ductal hyperplasia.

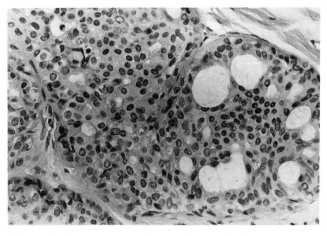

Figure 10.12. Atypical ductal hyperplasia.

11. Usual Hyperplasia and ADH vs Low-Grade DCIS

Our current definition of noncomedo DCIS requires that at least two membrane-lined spaces be occupied by a uniform population of cells having the structural characteristics of cribriform, micropapillary, or solid DCIS. The guidelines developed by Page require that ductal proliferative lesions lacking this fully developed, uniform population in two spaces be designated as ADH. Similarly, if a portion of a proliferation considered for a diagnosis of DCIS also includes a population of narrow, streaming, myoepithelial-like cells, the designation should be ADH. In the guidelines proposed by Tavassoli (1992), an overall size criterion of 2 mm is required for a diagnosis of DCIS. Lesions with histologic features of low-grade DCIS which measure less than 2 mm in the largest dimension are considered ADH.

It is well recognized that DCIS commonly arises within the setting of ADH. When ADH is present alone, it is most commonly a small lesion confined to a single duct and adjacent ductules.

To distinguish *usual hyperplasia* and *ADH* from *DCIS*, it is necessary to recognize the established features of each pattern of *low-grade DCIS* so that ADH, which falls short of these criteria, can be distinguished. Currently, it appears appropriate to observe the suggested size or space criterion when naming these lesions.

Low-grade cribriform DCIS is recognized when terminal duct lobular units are filled with a uniform cell population which is punctuated by crisp, punched-out spaces (Figs. 11.1–11.3). These spaces have a sieve-like arrangement and should be lined by uniform, somewhat squared-off cells similar to those found elsewhere in the duct. If the spaces are lined wholly or in part by spindly, longitudinally oriented cells, this is indicative of persisting myoepithelium and is typical of areas of ADH or of usual hyperplasia (Figs. 11.4–11.6) rather than DCIS. In low-grade DCIS lesions, it is common to identify residual myoepithelial cells arranged around the periphery of the duct space (Fig. 11.2); these cells, however, do not persist as part of the intraluminal proliferation in DCIS (Fig. 11.3). Myoepithelial cells are consistently present in the intraluminal proliferation of fenestrated usual hyperplasia (Figs. 11.4, 11.6).

The proliferation in low-grade cribriform DCIS commonly has crisp, punched-out spaces that often contain calcifications (Figs. 11.7, 11.8). When bars are present, they appear stiff and nontapering (Fig. 11.1). In some cases the central portion of the ductal space is empty,

and the cellular proliferation forms single or multitiered "Roman bridges" with rigid arches lacking spindly cells (Fig. 11.9). In some cases, the spaces in cribriform DCIS are less well developed and appear somewhat rosette-like in arrangement (Fig. 11.10). Cytologically, cribriform DCIS can often be distinguished from usual hyperplasia based on the presence of a monomorphic cell population and lack of myoepithelial cells within the proliferation (Figs. 11.11, 11.12).

The *micropapillary pattern* of low-grade DCIS must be distinguished from those cases of usual hyperplasia which have a micropapillary pattern (Fig. 11.13–11.15). Micropapillary DCIS is characterized by papillary excrescences which project into the lumina of the ducts or lobular spaces, have no fibrovascular cores, and are composed of uniform cells arranged like multiple peninsulas projecting into a space (Figs. 11.16–11.18). Sometimes necrosis of individual cells is present. The tips of the projections are often broad or bulbous in appearance (Fig. 11.19), and in many cases the micropapillary and cribriform patterns may coalesce (Figs. 11.20–11.22). In some instances, micropapillary DCIS has a higher nuclear grade and more necrosis (Figs. 11.23, 11.24). Recent studies indicate that this micropapillary pattern of DCIS tends to colonize extensively along the ductal and lobular units. If the atypical micropapillary proliferation of DCIS does not involve most of the circumference of the duct spaces or involves an area less than two spaces or measuring less than 2 mm, then this lesion should be designated as ADH with micropapillary features. Micropapillary hyperplasia of the usual type retains the double-cell population in both the micropapillary excrescences and surrounding proliferation (Fig. 11.14). The true papillary carcinomas, which have supporting fibrovascular cores, more commonly occur in larger ducts rather than terminal duct-lobular units and must be distinguished from large duct papillomas. This subject is discussed further in Section 4.

The *solid pattern* of low-grade DCIS is composed of a uniform population of neoplastic cells which is not interrupted by populations of swirling or spindling cells, as in usual hyperplasia (Figs. 11.25–11.27). Solid DCIS lacks significant necrosis (Figs. 11.28, 11.29). Occasionally, early organization toward a pattern of the cribriform type can be recognized within the solid growth pattern as a rosette-like arrangement of cells (Fig. 11.30). This early rosette pattern is also helpful in distinguishing solid-pattern DCIS from LCIS.

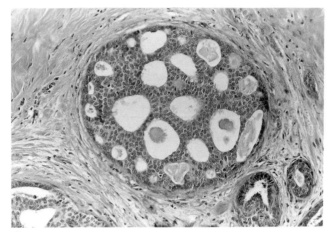

Figure 11.1. Cribriform intraductal carcinoma.

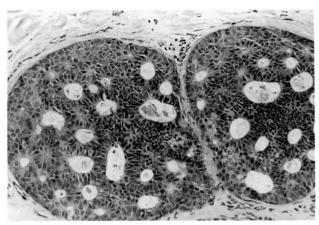

Figure 11.2. Cribriform intraductal carcinoma, intermediate grade.

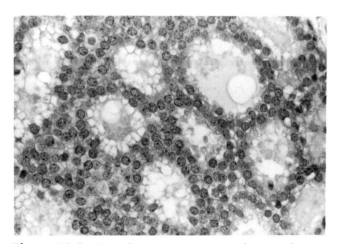

Figure 11.3. Ductal carcinoma in situ, low grade.

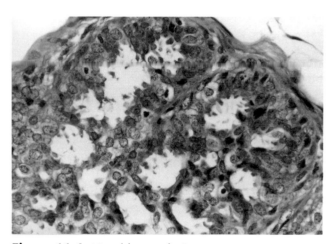

Figure 11.4. Usual hyperplasia.

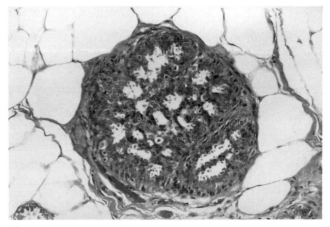

Figure 11.5. Usual hyperplasia.

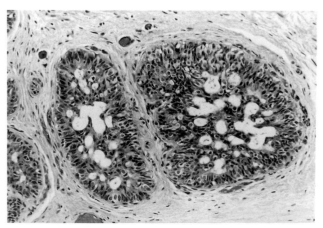

Figure 11.6. Usual hyperplasia.

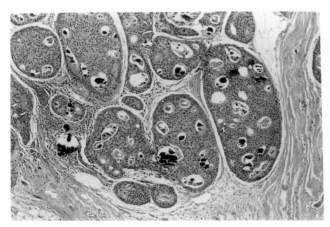

Figure 11.7. Ductal carcinoma in situ, low grade.

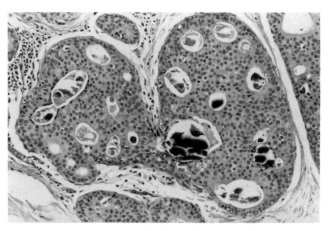

Figure 11.8. Ductal carcinoma in situ, low grade.

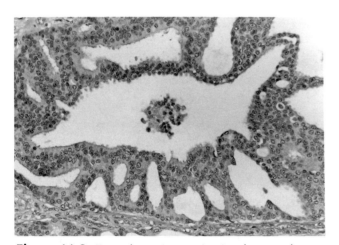

Figure 11.9. Ductal carcinoma in situ, low grade.

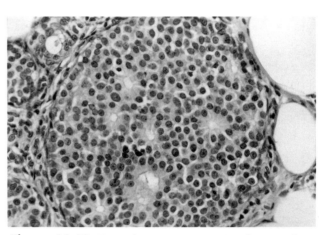

Figure 11.10. Ductal carcinoma in situ, low grade.

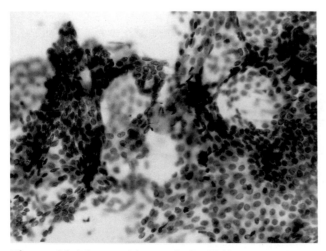

Figure 11.11. Usual hyperplasia. FNA.

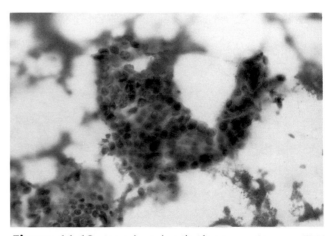

Figure 11.12. Intraductal cribriform carcinoma. FNA.

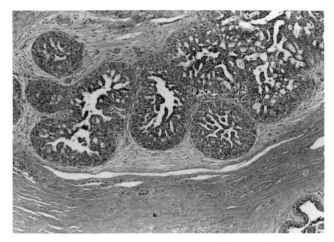

Figure 11.13. Micropapillary usual hyperplasia.

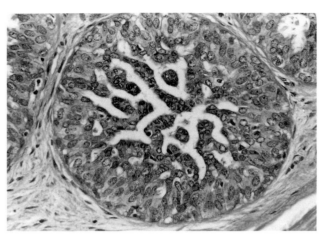

Figure 11.14. Micropapillary usual hyperplasia.

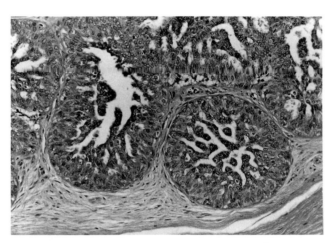

Figure 11.15. Micropapillary usual hyperplasia.

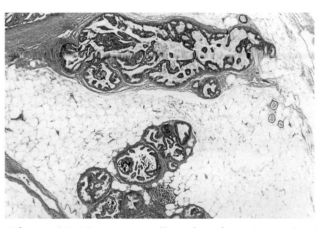

Figure 11.16. Micropapillary ductal carcinoma in situ.

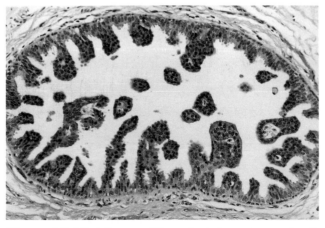

Figure 11.17. Micropapillary ductal carcinoma in situ.

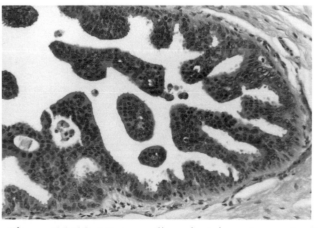

Figure 11.18. Micropapillary ductal carcinoma in situ.

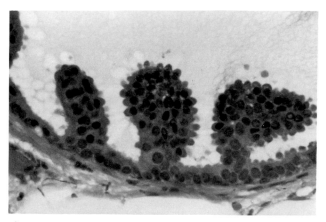

Figure 11.19. Micropapillary ductal carcinoma in situ.

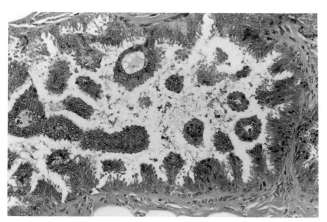

Figure 11.20. Micropapillary ductal carcinoma in situ.

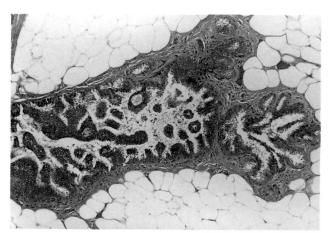

Figure 11.21. Micropapillary ductal carcinoma in situ.

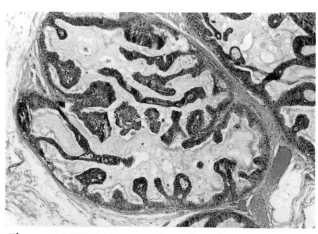

Figure 11.22. Micropapillary ductal carcinoma in situ.

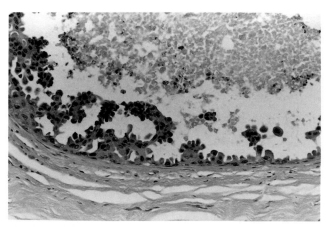

Figure 11.23. Micropapillary ductal carcinoma in situ.

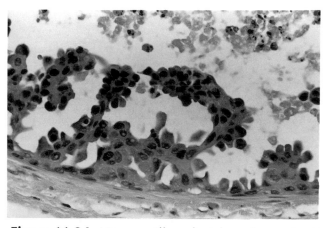

Figure 11.24. Micropapillary ductal carcinoma in situ.

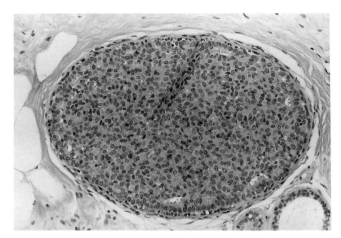

Figure 11.25. Solid usual hyperplasia.

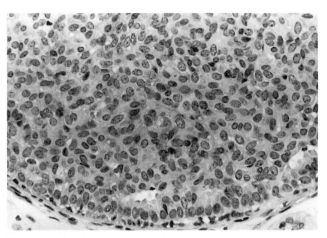

Figure 11.26. Solid usual hyperplasia.

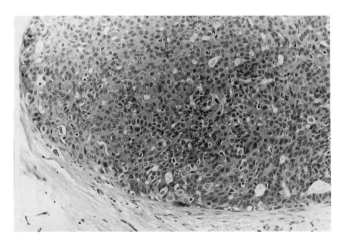

Figure 11.27. Solid usual hyperplasia.

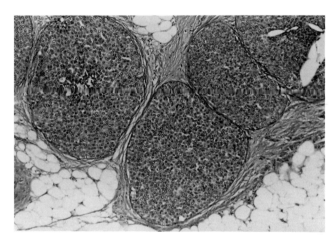

Figure 11.28. Solid ductal carcinoma in situ, low grade.

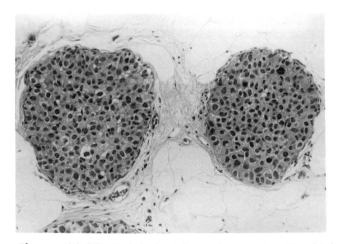

Figure 11.29. Solid ductal carcinoma in situ, high grade.

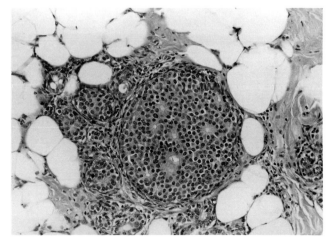

Figure 11.30. Solid ductal carcinoma in situ, low grade.

12. Low-Grade DCIS vs Intermediate and High-Grade DCIS

Recent studies have shown that evaluation of nuclear grade is more important in assessing the potential for recurrence of DCIS after inadequate excision than is the presence or absence of necrosis in the intraductal proliferation.

The classic example of *high-grade DCIS* is the comedo variant, characterized by a solid growth pattern of anaplastic carcinoma cells associated with central comedo necrosis which is commonly calcified (Figs. 12.1, 12.2). This comedo pattern of DCIS characteristically extends from the terminal ducts into contiguous lobular units, often distending them so that they resemble small ducts. High-grade comedo DCIS of this type is commonly associated with periductal fibrosis, so that a density or mass effect may be imaged radiographically or even palpated in extensive lesions. Comedo DCIS, like other types of high-grade DCIS, is often associated with a periductal lymphocytic inflammatory reaction. The linear, branching pattern of calcification produced by comedo carcinoma as it ramifies through ducts and lobules produces a characteristic mammographic pattern that is almost pathognomonic of this disorder.

A second pattern of *high-grade DCIS* is characterized by ducts lined by high-grade anaplastic cells which undergo necrosis and sloughing to create a pseudopapillary pattern (Fig. 12.3) similar to that of micropapillary DCIS.

In this lesion, necrosis is present but often does not produce the accumulated central debris that is characteristic of the classic comedo pattern. This high-grade pseudopapillary lesion must be distinguished from the more characteristic low-grade micropapillary DCIS lesion (Fig. 12.4), which may have focal necrosis and desquamation of papillae but does not have the large anaplastic cell population which designates high-grade DCIS.

Intermediate- and *high-grade DCIS* may demonstrate features of cribriform DCIS, which is characterized by higher-grade cells and usually by necrosis. Nuclei show more nuclear pleomorphism and prominent nucleoli (Figs. 12.5–12.7). Other patterns of intermediate-grade DCIS have cribriform or fenestrated growth patterns, as in low-grade cribriform DCIS, but have larger cells, larger, more irregular nuclei, and a tendency to undergo necrosis (Fig. 12.8). Other intermediate- or high-grade patterns of DCIS may resemble solid low-grade DCIS but differ in having some central necrosis or variation in cell type, such as clear cell patterns (Fig. 12.9). Most of these patterns can be distinguished from low-grade DCIS (Figs. 12.10–12.12).

Since micropapillary DCIS may have necrosis even in low-grade lesions due to its delicate architectural pattern, it is often not practical to attempt to separate intermediate- and low-grade micropapillary carcinoma.

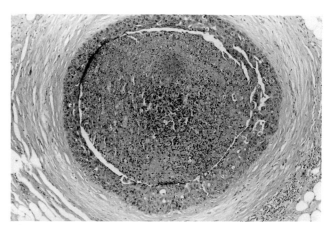

Figure 12.1. Comedo ductal carcinoma in situ.

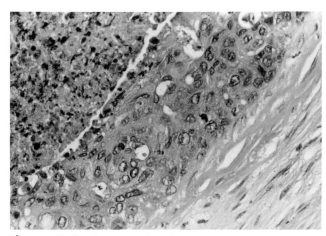

Figure 12.2. Comedo ductal carcinoma in situ.

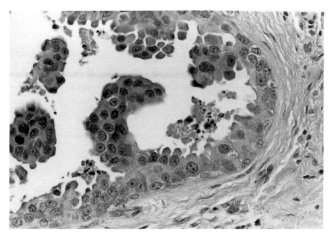

Figure 12.3. High-grade micropapillary ductal carcinoma in situ.

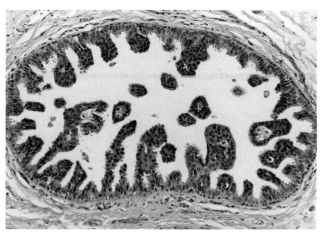

Figure 12.4. Low-grade micropapillary ductal carcinoma in situ.

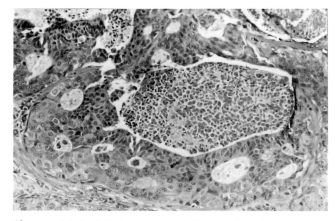

Figure 12.5. High-grade cribriform ductal carcinoma in situ.

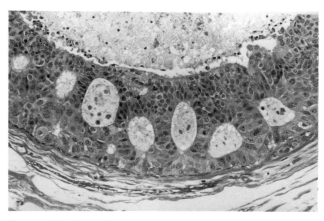

Figure 12.6. High-grade cribriform ductal carcinoma in situ.

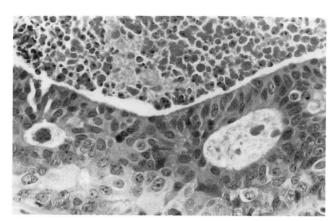

Figure 12.7. High-grade cribriform ductal carcinoma in situ.

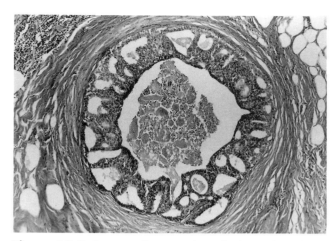

Figure 12.8. Intermediate-grade cribriform ductal carcinoma in situ.

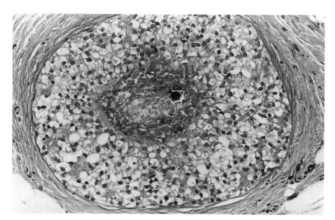

Figure 12.9. Clear cell comedo ductal carcinoma in situ.

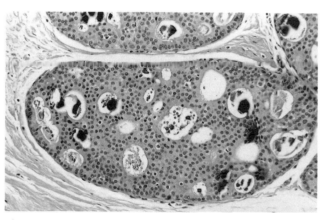

Figure 12.10. Low-grade cribriform ductal carcinoma in situ.

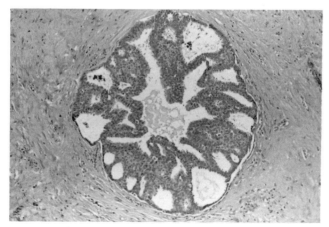

Figure 12.11. Low-grade cribriform ductal carcinoma in situ.

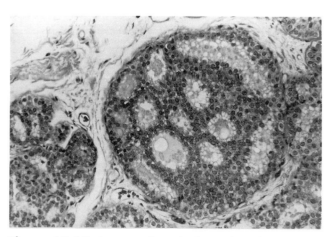

Figure 12.12. Low-grade cribriform ductal carcinoma in situ.

13. Cribriform DCIS vs Infiltrating Cribriform Carcinoma

Mammary lesions composed of uniform neoplastic cell aggregates with characteristic crisp, punched-out spaces are not always confined within the membranes of duct and lobular structures. Such *cribriform* nests of cells may be invasive (*infiltrating cribriform carcinoma*) (Fig. 13.1), a lesion recognized as a variant of well-differentiated infiltrating ductal carcinoma, with a good prognosis similar to that of the tubular type.

Distinction between infiltrating cribriform carcinoma and cribriform DCIS (Fig. 13.2) is best done by determining the presence or absence of residual basement membrane and peripheral myoepithelial cells that characterize the architecture of a "previously constructed" unit, i.e., the foundation membrane of the terminal duct-lobular unit. In lesions of *infiltrating cribriform carcinoma*, a careful search will fail to find residual myoepithelium, and the peripheral cells comprising the lesion will appear to be in direct contact with the connective tissue of the stroma of the breast (Fig. 13.3, 13.4). In contrast, low-grade *cribriform DCIS* nearly always has some identifiable remnant of the preexisting myoepithelium and basement membrane (Figs. 13.5, 13.6).

Infiltrating cribriform carcinoma is commonly associated with the single infiltrating gland structures of TC. In rare instances, the infiltrating cribriform glands are associated with vessel-rich stroma, hemorrhage, hemosiderin deposition, and multinucleated, osteoclast-like giant cells. These lesions are more specifically designated as *mammary carcinoma with stromal giant cells* (see also Section 5).

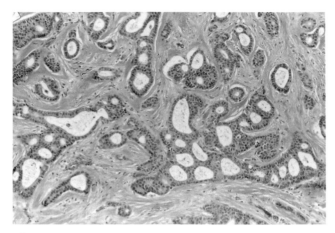

Figure 13.1. Infiltrating cribriform carcinoma.

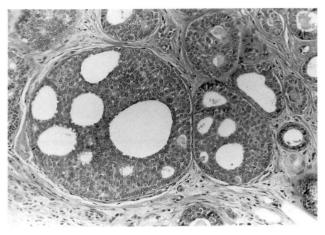

Figure 13.2. Cribriform ductal carcinoma in situ.

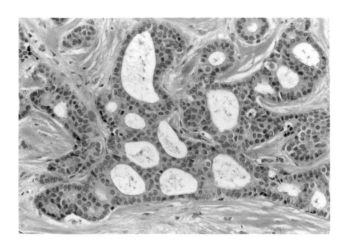

Figure 13.3. Infiltrating cribriform carcinoma.

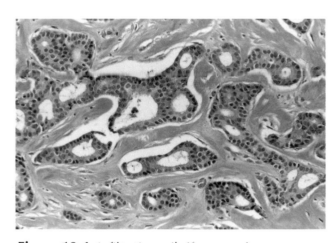

Figure 13.4. Infiltrating cribriform carcinoma.

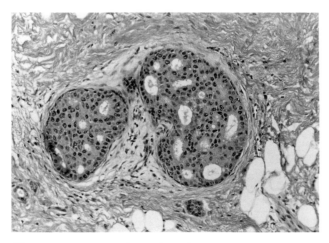

Figure 13.5. Cribriform ductal carcinoma in situ.

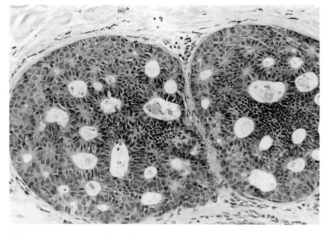

Figure 13.6. Cribriform ductal carcinoma in situ.

14. Apocrine Hyperplasia and Atypical Apocrine Hyperplasia vs Apocrine DCIS

Apocrine metaplasia in breast lesions has a very variable appearance. Since apocrine nuclei are usually large and typically contain prominent nucleoli, even innocuous metaplastic and hyperplastic apocrine lesions may have a worrisome appearance (Figs. 14.1–14.4). Nonproliferative but atypical-looking single-layered apocrine lesions having a three-fold variation in nuclear size are commonly designated *atypical apocrine metaplasia.* This atypical, nonproliferative pattern of apocrine cells is considered by many as a variant of little clinical significance.

Currently, there are no uniformly accepted criteria for identifying those atypical-looking apocrine lesions which have clinical significance. Recently, however, Tavassoli and Norris at the Armed Forces Institute of Pathology (AFIP) have presented a very detailed list of criteria for designating atypical apocrine hyperplasia and intraductal apocrine carcinoma (1994). These guidelines are adopted for the following descriptions.

Atypical apocrine hyperplasia must demonstrate some proliferative activity, not merely the presence of some atypical-looking cells occurring in a single layer. Two general patterns of atypical apocrine hyperplasia are recognized. The first has proliferation in the form of cell stratification, tufting, or papillae formation (Fig. 14.5). This pattern requires cellular atypia with a three-fold variation in nuclear size and usually has prominent nucleoli.

The second recognized pattern of atypical apocrine hyperplasia includes apocrine proliferations with traditional atypical epithelial bridging patterns, including cribriform and arcade patterns which are often incomplete in that the entire ductal space is not completely involved by the proliferation (Fig. 14.6). This pattern of atypical apocrine hyperplasia, however, is not characterized by significantly atypical cells. The cytologic changes are characteristically mild and may consist only of an increased nuclear/cytoplasmic ratio. (The combination of cribriform pattern with marked atypia is placed in the intraductal carcinoma category rather than ADH). Some experts would also place the low nuclear grade cribriform pattern in the DCIS category, particularly if the cribriform pattern involves the whole circumference of the ductal space. Lesions of this type which exceed 2 mm in aggregate diameter should probably be designated as intraductal carcinoma.

Apocrine DCIS as designated by the AFIP group, has several different forms. The most common pattern is characterized by intraluminal necrosis and is designated as the *comedo (necrotic) type* (Figs. 14.7–14.9). In this pattern there are single or multiple layers of apocrine cells having moderate to marked cytologic atypia along with intraluminal necrosis. This pattern includes no size requirement and may be diagnosed when only a single ductule is involved.

The second pattern of intraductal apocrine carcinoma is the *noncomedo (nonnecrotic) type.* The *low-grade* form of this pattern is characterized by solid sheets of abnormal apocrine cells with a monotonous, uniform appearance (Figs. 14.10, 14.11) involving one or more ductal spaces with an aggregate dimension of >2 mm (all pathologists do not agree on size requirements). *Intermediate-grade noncomedo apocrine* DCIS is characterized by more severe atypia and distinct cell borders having a solid, cribriform, or, rarely, papillary pattern (Fig. 14.12).

The third form of intraductal apocrine carcinoma designated by the AFIP group is very rare, consisting of true *papillary* apocrine lesions having delicate fibrovascular stalks and no myoepithelial cells. The relatively uniform atypical apocrine cells in the lesion grow in layers and form varying arcade and bridging patterns. This entity is discussed further in Section 4.

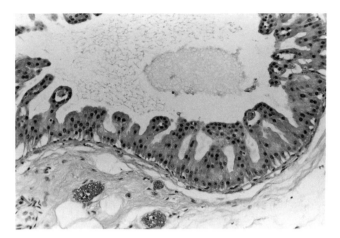

Figure 14.1. Apocrine hyperplasia.

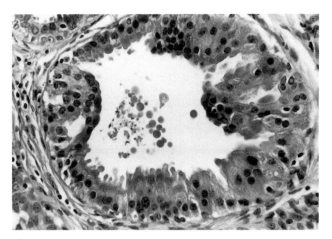

Figure 14.2. Apocrine hyperplasia.

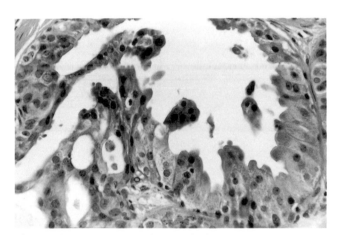

Figure 14.3. Apocrine hyperplasia.

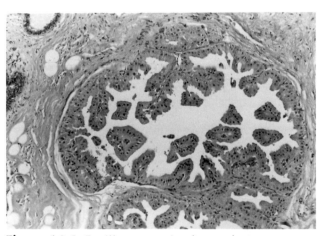

Figure 14.4. Papillary apocrine hyperplasia.

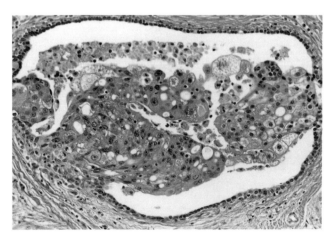

Figure 14.5. Atypical apocrine hyperplasia.

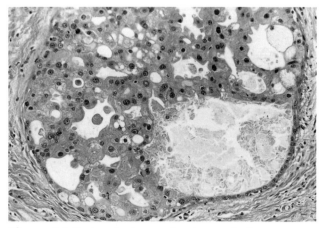

Figure 14.6. Atypical apocrine hyperplasia.

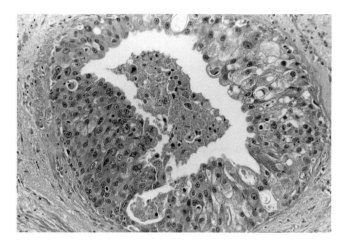

Figure 14.7. Apocrine ductal carcinoma in situ.

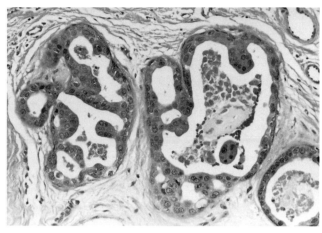

Figure 14.8. Apocrine ductal carcinoma in situ.

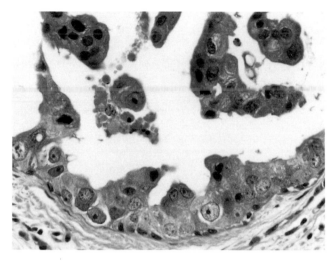

Figure 14.9. Apocrine ductal carcinoma in situ.

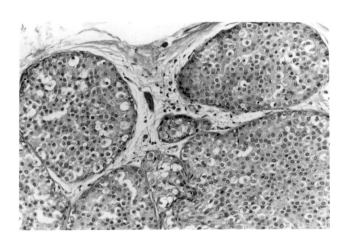

Figure 14.10. Apocrine ductal carcinoma in situ.

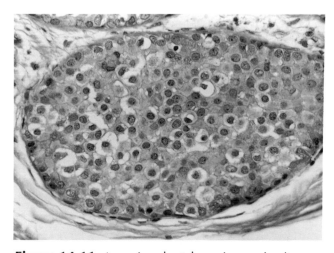

Figure 14.11. Apocrine ductal carcinoma in situ.

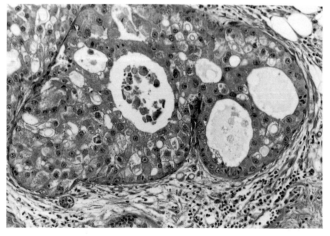

Figure 14.12. Apocrine ductal carcinoma in situ.

15. Usual Lobular Hyperplasia and ALH vs LCIS

The ductules distended by *usual hyperplasia* demonstrate the same cytologic features and patterns seen in ducts with usual hyperplasia (see Chapter 10). The membrane-bound spaces contain a cellular proliferation which includes cells of varying morphologic appearance, at least one of which resembles the myoepithelium. The nuclear shape and orientation are irregular, and the cell borders appear indistinct.

ALH indicates the emergence of the cell of lobular neoplasia within the terminal ductal lobular unit. The characteristic neoplastic cell is usually first recognized within the lobule as a monomorphic population of cells with round, clear, or pink-staining cytoplasm and round, bland nuclei commonly having small nucleoli (Fig. 15.1). The monomorphic cells of *lobular neoplasia* appear small but are often larger than the normal cellular components of the lobule. They never appear spindly. The cells are classically "loosely cohesive," but this arrangement appears to vary with fixation and processing artifact (Fig. 15.2). The cytoplasm of lobular neoplasia cells commonly demonstrate variably sized lumina which may contain secretory mucin droplets (Fig. 15.3), which stain positively with PAS after diastase digestion with mucicarmine and Alcian blue.

As lobular spaces become colonized by new cells in ALH, the neoplastic cell appears to gently push the normal or usual cells aside or lift them up as the new proliferating cells become more numerous (Fig. 15.3). The monomorphic cell population in ALH may extend into adjacent terminal ducts in a "pagetoid" fashion.

The difference between *ALH* and *LCIS* is one of degree. The criteria for distinction between these entities are not uniformly agreed on, but essentially they depend on how completely lobular units are filled and perhaps distended by the characteristic monomorphic cells of lobular neoplasia. Lobules which are filled or predominantly occupied by the cells of lobular neopla-

sia are designated as *LCIS* (Figs. 15.4–15.6), while those whose units contain fewer cells are called *ALH*. Pagetoid extension of the process into the adjacent terminal ducts, although more common in LCIS, may occur in both ALH and LCIS and cannot be used to distinguish between them.

The relevance of the distinction between LCIS and ALH has been demonstrated in several studies. These studies reveal that the subsequent development of invasive mammary carcinoma occurs approximately twice as often in women with prior biopsies demonstrating LCIS than in those whose prior biopsies demonstrated only ALH.

The Page criteria for *LCIS* require that at least half of the ductules in the lobular unit be completely filled, distorted, and distended with the characteristic cells of lobular neoplasia, so that no residual intercellular lumina exist. *ALH* should be diagnosed when a neoplastic cell population is present but fails to produce complete filling and distention of lobular units in over 50% of the ductules within a lobular unit (Fig. 15.2).

More recently, Rosen and Oberman have proposed less stringent criteria for a diagnosis of *LCIS*. Although they require that a lobule be predominantly filled by the neoplastic cells to earn a designation of LCIS, they do not require lobular distention or the total absence of gland lumina. While some authorities require involvement of two lobules for LCIS, Rosen and Oberman require only one.

The classic cell of LCIS is usually characterized as small, round, and containing a cytologically bland nucleus. In some cases, however, the neoplastic cells demonstrate considerable cytologic pleomorphism, and more varied appearance with larger pleomorphic nuclei with nucleoli *(pleomorphic variant of lobular carcinoma)*. Cytoplasmic vacuoles containing mucin are usually present in both types.

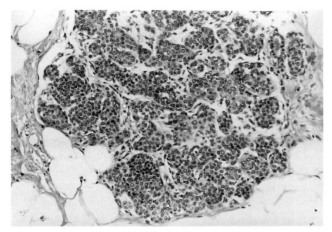

Figure 15.1. Atypical lobular hyperplasia.

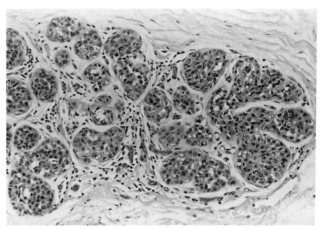

Figure 15.2. Atypical lobular hyperplasia.

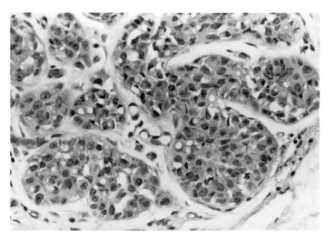

Figure 15.3. Atypical lobular hyperplasia.

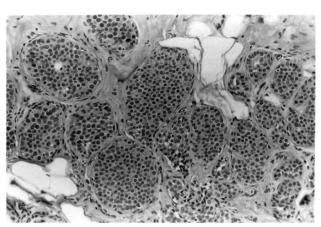

Figure 15.4. Lobular carcinoma in situ.

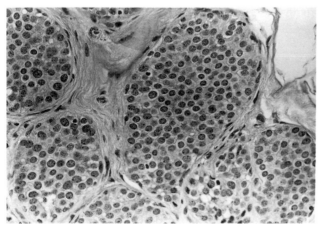

Figure 15.5. Lobular carcinoma in situ.

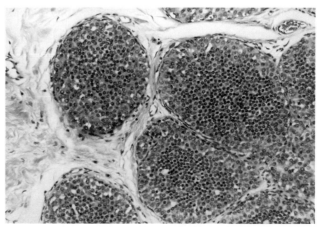

Figure 15.6. Lobular carcinoma in situ.

16. Lobular Extension of DCIS vs Ductal Extension of LCIS

Distinction between *LCIS* and colonization of lobules with *DCIS* may be difficult, particularly when one of the classic patterns of DCIS is not present in the adjacent terminal duct. Often, some suggestion of small secondary spaces or rosette patterns may be present which help to identify the lesion in the lobule as an extension of DCIS (Figs. 16.1–16.3). Otherwise, the pathologist must distinguish LCIS from DCIS on the basis of cytologic features. The presence of marked nuclear pleomorphism, very large cells, or small collections of necrotic cells usually indicate that a lesion represents lobular extension of DCIS (Figs. 16.4–16.6). Occasionally, however, necrotic cells may be seen in lesions of lobular neoplasia, and the pleomorphic variant of LCIS is associated with larger nuclei with less characteristic features.

On occasions where the distinction is between LCIS and a low-grade, solid type of DCIS within a lobule, it is usually most helpful to seek the cytologic features of lobular neoplasia. These include a tendency toward poor cell cohesion and the presence of small, round intracytoplasmic lumina which contain droplets of mucin. *LCIS* commonly extends into adjacent terminal ducts. The diagnosis of LCIS is made by identifying the cells of lobular neoplasia accumulating within lobular units. Cells of this same morphologic type may extend into extralobular terminal ducts and characteristically produces the pattern named *pagetoid spread* (Fig. 16.7). In pagetoid spread, the cells of lobular neoplasia appear to slide between the normal epithelial and myoepithelial cells of the terminal duct wall. Characteristically, the persisting normal epithelial cell component may appear focally flattened or compressed over the nests of neoplastic cells (Fig. 16.8).

It is important to remember that a diagnosis of LCIS cannot be made solely on the basis of pagetoid spread within the terminal duct. ALH also colonizes the duct in an identical, if somewhat subdued, fashion. The distinction between ALH and LCIS must rest on the degree of monomorphism and distention of the ductules of the lobule.

In distinguishing ductal involvement by *LCIS* from *DCIS*, several parameters should be considered. First, the neoplastic cell population must be right for LCIS. The cells should appear monomorphic, with round or oval clear or pink-staining cytoplasm surrounding relatively bland nuclei with small nucleoli (Fig. 16.7). Intracytoplasmic lumina are commonly identified in some of the cells. Second, the pattern should be consistent with those recognized for ductal extension of LCIS. This is most commonly pagetoid, although in more advanced lesions the clustered patterns may be lost. Cell necrosis generally militates against a diagnosis of LCIS, as does any tendency toward rosette formation, cribriform space formation, or papillary growth. Solid filling of the duct suggests the solid variant of DCIS if the cells do not exhibit cytoplasmic lumina.

Occasionally, the extralobular terminal duct has previously undergone hyperplastic proliferation and then secondarily becomes colonized by the neoplastic cells of *LCIS*. In this case, the neoplastic cells may grow over and around the benign proliferation, assuming the contours of the hyperplasia, or may accumulate as solid masses of cells peripheral to the hyperplastic lesion (Figs. 16.9, 16.10). *DCIS* may also extend along adjacent ductal passages and colonize lesions of usual hyperplasia (Figs. 16.11, 16.12).

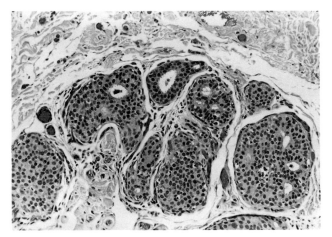

Figure 16.1. Low-grade ductal carcinoma in situ in the lobule.

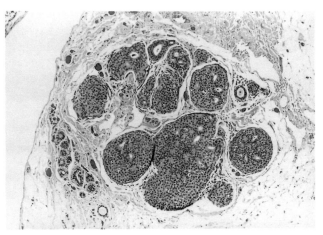

Figure 16.2. Low-grade ductal carcinoma in situ in the lobule.

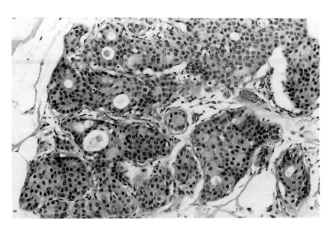

Figure 16.3. Low-grade ductal carcinoma in situ in the lobule.

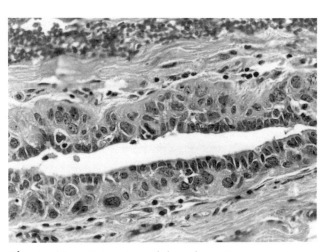

Figure 16.4. Extension of ductal carcinoma in situ.

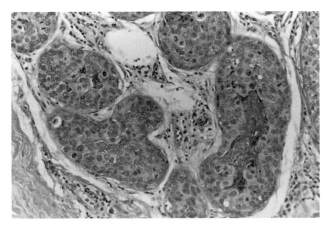

Figure 16.5. High-grade ductal carcinoma in situ in the lobule.

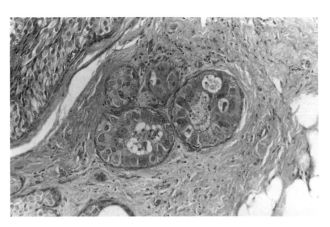

Figure 16.6. High-grade ductal carcinoma in situ in the lobule.

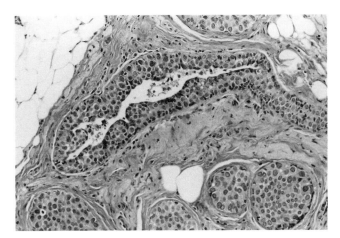

Figure 16.7. Lobular carcinoma in situ with duct extension.

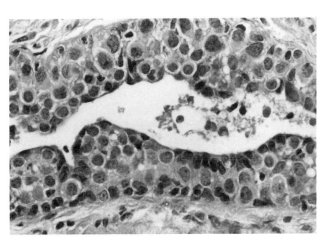

Figure 16.8. Lobular carcinoma in situ in pagetoid spread.

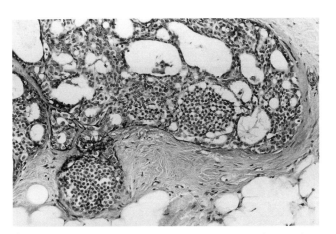

Figure 16.9. Lobular carcinoma in situ in hyperplasia.

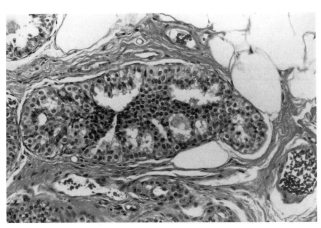

Figure 16.10. Lobular carcinoma in situ in hyperplasia.

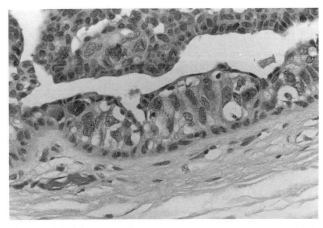

Figure 16.11. Ductal carcinoma in situ in hyperplasia.

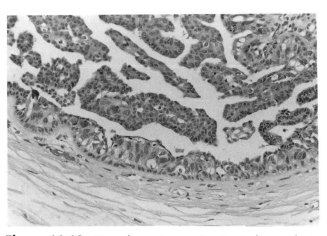

Figure 16.12. Ductal carcinoma in situ in hyperplasia.

17. Collagenous Spherulosis vs Cribriform DCIS and Adenoid Cystic Carcinoma

Collagenous spherulosis is an incidental microscopic finding within ductules which may occur in association with usual hyperplasia. The acellular spherules occur within secondary spaces and vary in size from approximately 20 to 100 μm in diameter. They may be few or many, and are always associated with an intraluminal proliferation of epithelial and myoepithelial cells similar to those of usual hyperplasia (Figs. 17.1–17.3). The spherules are predominantly collagen but also contain variable amounts of PAS-positive basement membrane–like material. The cells immediately adjacent to the spherules demonstrate a positive reaction to actin. They are believed to be myoepithelial cells and are responsible for secretion of the collagenous material.

Collagenous spherulosis must be differentiated from low-grade *cribriform DCIS,* which at low power also produces the impression of round, punched-out spaces (Fig. 17.4). At high power, however, the cell prolifera-

tion of collagenous spherulosis is seen as spindly and partially myoepithelial in nature (Fig. 17.2), while the DCIS pattern is recognized as monomorphic. Similarly, with special stains, the spaces in collagenous spherulosis can be identified as containing solid connective tissue rather than empty spaces.

A significant consideration in the histologic differential diagnosis of collagenous spherulosis is *adenoid cystic carcinoma* because the hyaline spherules of both lesions are similar in appearance (Figs. 17.5, 17.6). Adenoid cystic carcinoma of the breast is an invasive lesion characteristically associated with a mass. It is composed of two cell types (a basaloid cell population which predominates and a smaller population of cells with eosinophilic cytoplasm). By contrast, collagenous spherulosis is always a microscopic finding associated with hyperplasia in mammary ductules, and it lacks the invasive two-cell type growth pattern of adenoid cystic carcinoma.

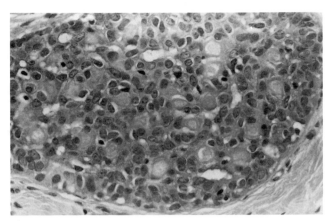

Figure 17.1. Collagenous spherulosis.

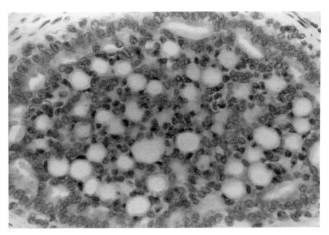

Figure 17.2. Collagenous spherulosis.

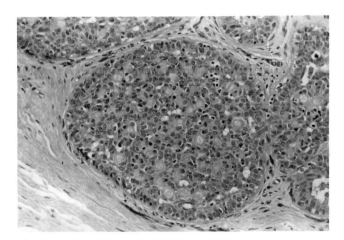

Figure 17.3. Collagenous spherulosis.

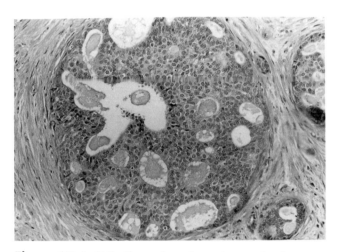

Figure 17.4. Cribriform ductal carcinoma in situ.

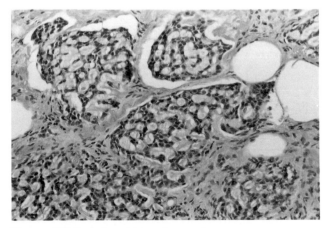

Figure 17.5. Adenoid cystic carcinoma.

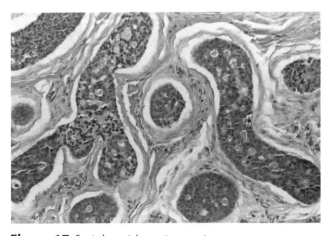

Figure 17.6. Adenoid cystic carcinoma.

Section 3

RADIAL SCARS, RADIAL SCLEROSING LESIONS, AND COMPLEX SCLEROSING LESIONS

GENERAL CONSIDERATIONS

Radial sclerosing lesions are distinctive benign epithelial proliferations associated with central fibrous cores and a radiating or spiculated periphery that may mimic carcinoma radiographically and occasionally grossly. Since the central core often contains trapped ductular or tubular structures, the lesion is often a difficult diagnostic problem histologically and must be distinguished from infiltrating carcinoma, particularly TC. In addition, the occasional replacement or colonization of the benign epithelial structure by atypical intraductal lesions requires further diagnostic discrimination.

The best early description and illustrations of radial sclerosing lesions were given by Fenoglio and Lattes in 1974, using the term *sclerosing papillary proliferation.* Subsequently, the term *radial scar* became widely used by both pathologists and radiologists and has been endorsed by Tavassoli (1992) and by Page and Anderson (for lesions less than 1 cm). The latter authors have encouraged the use of *complex sclerosing lesion* for lesions greater than 1 cm. Recently, Rosen and Oberman have recommended the term *radial sclerosing lesion* for all such lesions, commenting that the postinflammatory pathogenesis of the lesion is unproved and that their term describes the configuration of the process histologically and mammographically, while being sufficiently nonspecific to encompass the broad range of microscopic components encountered in these lesions. Although we generally use the term *radial scar* in our own practice, the newer term *radial sclerosing lesion* will be used in the chapters concerning differential diagnosis.

IMAGING

Most radial sclerosing lesions appear as areas of architectural distortion on a mammogram, and these images may appear spiculated. These lesions are more likely to have an area of radiolucency near the center, perhaps due to entrapment of adipose tissue within the scar; however, this finding is not always reliable and may be seen in both carcinomas and scars. The presence of microcalcifications exclusively within a spiculated density is more commonly associated with carcinoma than with radial sclerosing lesions.

GROSS

Most small radial sclerosing lesions are probably not easily observed grossly, but are discovered histologically when mammographically directed biopsies are done for distortion or small, spiculated lesions. Many are found only as incidental lesions on microscopy. Larger lesions, or smaller ones which are expected and carefully looked for, usually appear as an irregular density with a white, fibrous center having narrow spicules or bands of fibrous tissue which radiate peripherally into the fat. If chalky streaks (reflecting elastosis in the lesion) are prominent, the tumor may strongly resemble an infiltrating carcinoma.

18. Radial Sclerosing Lesions vs Infiltrating Carcinoma

Although the infiltrative appearance of the tubules in the midst of *radial sclerosing lesions* mimics *infiltrating carcinoma*, satisfactory differentiation of these lesions requires examination of both the peripheral and central areas of suspicious-looking sclerosing lesions. The periphery typically contains areas of adenosis, usual ductal hyperplasia, or both (Figs. 18.1, 18.2). When ductal hyperplasia is present, it is commonly papillary and in fact may be a papilloma. Analysis of these areas then follows the usual criteria for distinguishing among adenosis, hyperplasia, and papillomas (see Sections 1, 2, and 4) based on structural and cytologic features. The most important feature is always the demonstration of myoepithelial cells within the hyperplastic proliferations and at the periphery of the ductules of adenosis.

The distinction between benign radial sclerosing lesions and infiltrating carcinoma is usually most difficult in the central portion of the scar. Regardless of their etiology, benign *radial sclerosing lesions* appear entrapped, as if small ductules were caught in the midst of a scarring process and somehow managed to survive (Figs. 18.3, 18.4). The ductules appear somewhat atrophic or pinched and are usually wrapped in dense collagenous tissue. To prove the benign nature of such a lesion, residual myoepithelia at the periphery of these structures must be demonstrated (Figs. 18.5, 18.6). Myoepithelial cells may appear spindly or as small, round nuclei with variably sized, clear cytoplasm. In some single ductal structures, only one or two myoepithelial cells may be found; however, this may be adequate if other, more convincing ducts are present. In

general, once a majority of the structures are found to include myoepithelial cells and the group of ducts all appear similar or of the same kind, the occasional absence of these cells is permitted. In the experience of most pathologists, the emergence of invasive TC from the center of an otherwise typical benign radial sclerosing lesion is extremely unusual. In difficult cases, immunohistochemical markers such as actin may be used to accentuate the myoepithelial cells.

Infiltrating carcinoma, in contrast, does not have myoepithelial cells (Figs. 18.7–18.9). The tubules of well-differentiated infiltrating duct carcinomas, particularly TC, have low-grade nuclei and are characteristically lined by one or two cell layers, all of which are the same cell types (Figs. 18.10, 18.11). The tubules of infiltrating carcinoma often appear to be in direct contact with the stroma and not enveloped by bands of collagen. Infiltrating TC commonly invades adjacent fat in a vigorous fashion (Figs. 18.8, 18.9), whereas the tubular structures of benign radial sclerosing lesions typically appear relatively atrophic and are limited to the scarred areas of stroma (Fig. 18.12). Low-grade DCIS is commonly present adjacent to TC (Fig. 18.9).

The stroma in the central zones of benign sclerosing lesions typically consists of both collagen and elastic tissue. The collagen is usually dense and poorly cellular, and the elastic tissue is characteristically amorphous (Figs. 18.5, 18.6). This type of elastic tissue accumulation may be very similar to that which occurs in infiltrating carcinoma and should not influence the differential diagnosis.

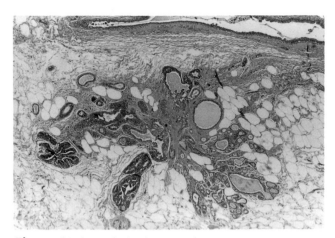

Figure 18.1. Radial sclerosing lesion.

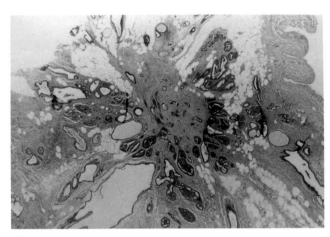

Figure 18.2. Radial sclerosing lesion.

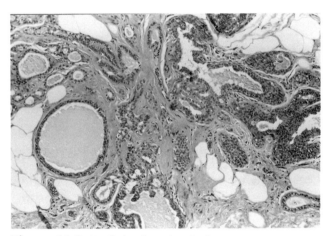

Figure 18.3. Radial sclerosing lesion.

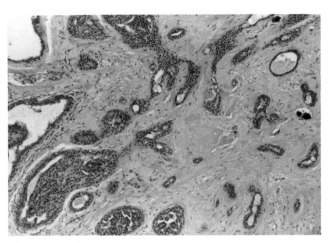

Figure 18.4. Radial sclerosing lesion.

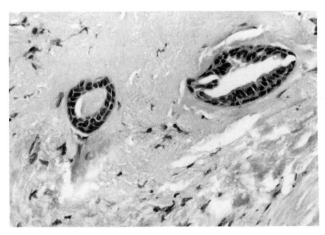

Figure 18.5. Radial sclerosing lesion.

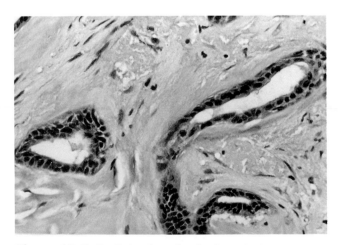

Figure 18.6. Radial sclerosing lesion.

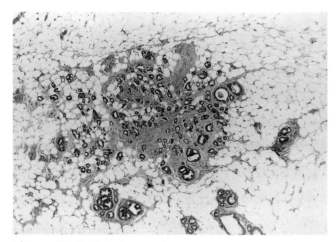

Figure 18.7. Tubular carcinoma.

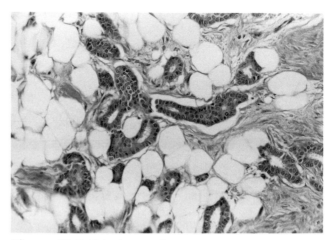

Figure 18.8. Tubular carcinoma.

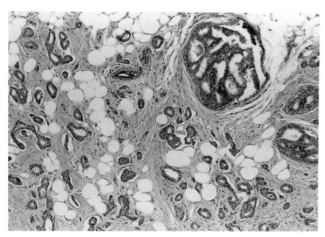

Figure 18.9. Tubular carcinoma with low-grade ductal carcinoma in situ.

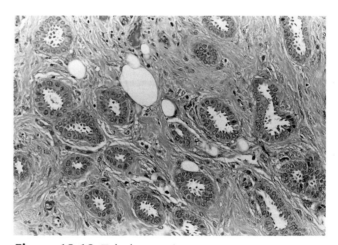

Figure 18.10. Tubular carcinoma.

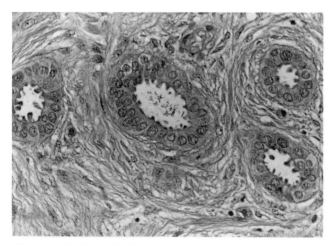

Figure 18.11. Tubular carcinoma.

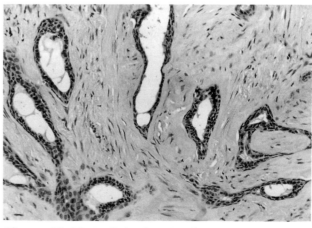

Figure 18.12. Radial sclerosing lesion.

19. DCIS and ADH within Radial Sclerosing Lesions vs Usual Radial Scars and Infiltrating Carcinoma

Low-grade DCIS, particularly with cribriform or micropapillary patterns, may ramify extensively within ducts and lobular units. Occasionally, it may also undergo a sclerosing process resulting in radial sclerosing lesions in which entrapment of DCIS may be difficult to distinguish from *usual radial scars* and sometimes from infiltrating carcinoma. In cases where the radial sclerosing lesion is entirely of the *usual* type (Figs. 19.1, 19.2), the peripheral proliferative lesion demonstrates the typical features of adenosis (Fig. 19.3), usual hyperplasia (Fig. 19.4), or papilloma. In these cases, the central entrapped ductules may demonstrate remnants of non-atypical proliferative activity and are always enclosed by myoepithelium (Fig. 19.5). The accumulation of a monomorphic cell population within such proliferations (Fig. 19.6) is suggestive of atypical ductal hyperplasia or a near-by intraductal carcinoma.

In *radial sclerosing lesions having DCIS,* the peripheral unsclerosed areas contain terminal ducts and ductules filled with varying degrees of ADH and non-comedo DCIS (Figs. 19.7, 19.8). This presence of ADH and DCIS peripheral to zones of sclerosis obviously creates strong suspicion that the central areas are invasive. Caution is well advised since this is the environ-ment where infiltrating TC or similar low-grade tumors, such as invasive cribriform carcinoma, may arise.

Some pathologists tend to overcall such "entrapped" areas of DCIS, and it is important to apply strict criteria to establish the differential diagnosis between DCIS which has sclerosed (Figs. 19.9, 19.10) and an *infiltrating carcinoma* which is actually invading the mammary stroma. As in all sclerosing lesions, the persistence of some myoepithelial cells is key to the distinction (Figs. 19.9, 19.11). Virtually all ADH lesions retain a generous population of myoepithelium at the periphery of the membrane-bound space, and most examples of low-grade DCIS retain varying amounts of the original myoepithelial population adjacent to the outer membrane. This myoepithelial cell population is retained in the radial sclerosing lesions of DCIS and ADH (Figs. 19.6, 19.11) and allows the pathologist to avoid overcalling such lesions as infiltrating tubular or cribriform carcinoma which should have no myoepithelial population, (Fig. 19.12). Similarly, "entrapped," DCIS may be wrapped in thickened bands of collagen (Fig. 19.10), and this may help distinguish noninvasive lesions from the brisk desmoplastic fibrosis associated with some infiltrating carcinomas.

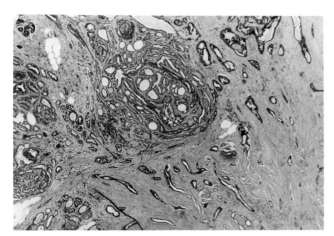

Figure 19.1. Radial sclerosing lesion.

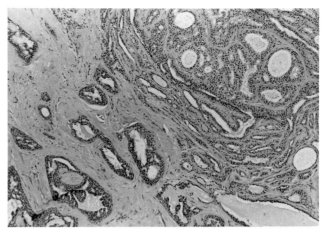

Figure 19.2. Radial sclerosing lesion.

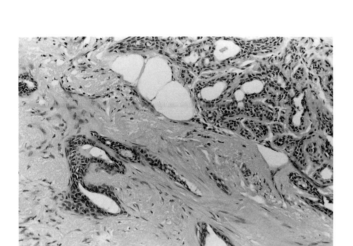

Figure 19.3. Radial sclerosing lesion.

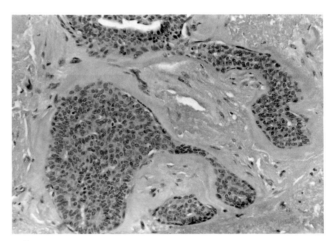

Figure 19.4. Radial sclerosing lesion.

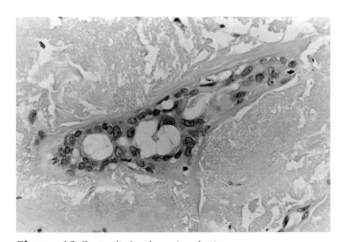

Figure 19.5. Radial sclerosing lesion.

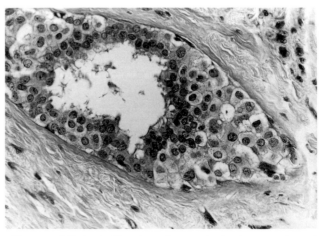

Figure 19.6. Infiltrating hyperplasia in a sclerosing lesion.

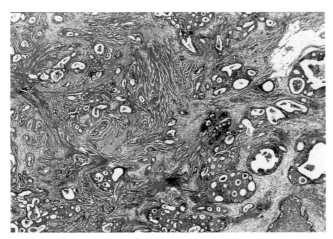

Figure 19.7. Ductal carcinoma in situ in a sclerosing lesion.

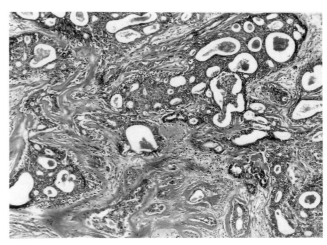

Figure 19.8. Ductal carcinoma in situ in a sclerosing lesion.

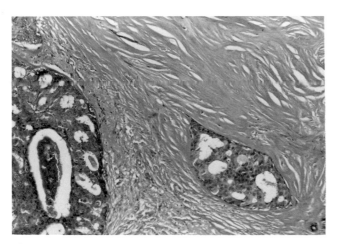

Figure 19.9. Ductal carcinoma in situ in a sclerosing lesion.

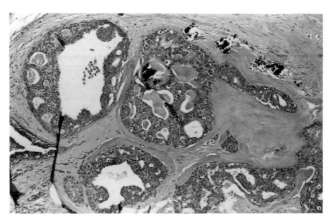

Figure 19.10. Ductal carcinoma in situ in a sclerosing lesion.

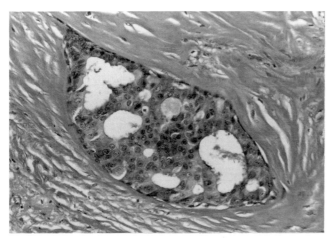

Figure 19.11. Ductal carcinoma in situ in a sclerosing lesion.

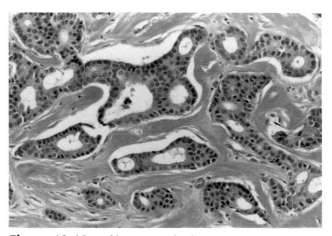

Figure 19.12. Infiltrating cribriform carcinoma.

20. LCIS and ALH in Radial Sclerosing Lesions vs Infiltrating Carcinoma

Radial sclerosing lesions commonly have areas of adenosis at their periphery, as well as trapped adenosis within the central scar (Figs. 20.1, 20.2), and these may become colonized by the cells of lobular neoplasia. As with ALH and LCIS in other locations, the process becomes recognized as the ductules within the lobules of adenosis become filled and perhaps distended by the characteristic monomorphic cell population of lobular neoplasia (Fig. 20.3). The abnormal cell population may also be present in the narrowed, sclerosed, or trapped ductules of the central scarred zone of the sclerosing lesion and create the appearance of a true *infiltrating carcinoma* (Fig. 20.4). The distinction between trapped LCIS and true invasive carcinoma requires the demonstration of myoepithelial cells, at least focally, at the periphery of the pseudoinfiltrating ductular structures (Fig. 20.4). Myoepithelial cells may vary in this lesion, appearing either spindly or round and lymphocyte-like, but they are usually distinguishable from the larger round to oval cells of lobular neoplasia. An immunohistochemical stain for actin may be helpful in identifying myoepithelial cells. The pathologist should not make a diagnosis of invasive lobular carcinoma unless clear-cut "unenveloped" stromal invasion is documented, either in the classic linear infiltration (Indian-file) pattern or with groups of cells that infiltrate stroma (Fig. 20.5).

As with all radial sclerosing patterns, the relationship between the infiltrative or pseudoinfiltrative ductules and the adjacent adipose tissue must be carefully evaluated. In general, benign radial sclerosing patterns have tubules embedded in an elastic and collagenous matrix or scar (Figs. 20.1, 20.2), and these do not invade directly into fatty stromal tissue. When radial sclerosing lesions do contain an in situ component of either the ductal or lobular type or areas of atypical hyperplasia (Fig. 20.6), additional levels or deeper sections should be taken from the paraffin block so that legitimate areas of invasion will not be missed. In obtaining additional sections from suspicious lesions, it is often best to start with a few gentle serial sections lest the lesion disappear too quickly.

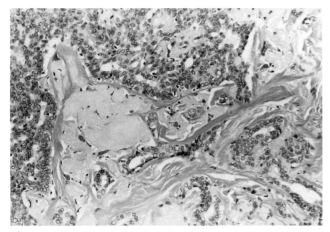

Figure 20.1. Radial sclerosing lesion.

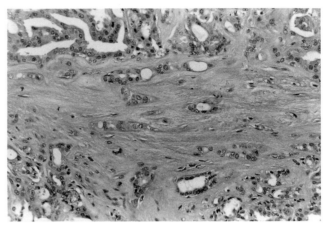

Figure 20.2. Sclerosing lesion with apocrine cells.

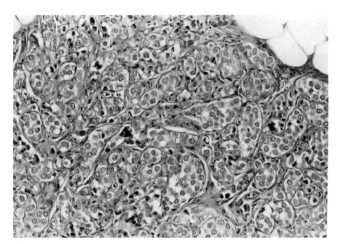

Figure 20.3. Lobular neoplasia in adenosis.

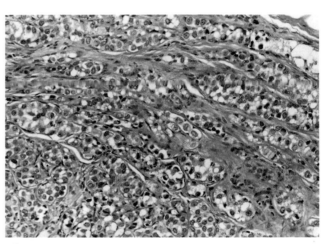

Figure 20.4. Lobular neoplasia in a sclerosing lesion.

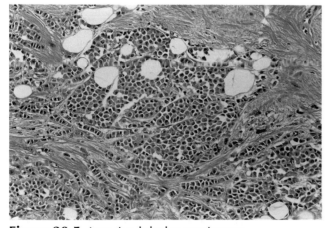

Figure 20.5. Invasive lobular carcinoma.

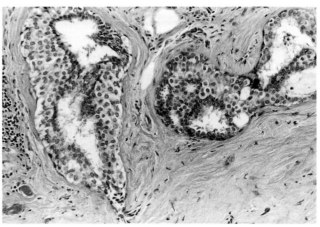

Figure 20.6. Atypical hyperplasia in a sclerosing lesion.

21. Postbiopsy and Traumatic Alterations in In Situ Carcinoma vs Infiltrating Carcinoma

Remote biopsy sites with mature fibrous scar tissue are generally not diagnostic problems. However, they may present the same differential diagnostic features discussed in Chapter 19 on DCIS lesions and radial scars.

The most common *postbiopsy problems* currently encountered occur in DCIS lesions which have been recently aspirated by FNA or core biopsy. In these needle biopsies, terminal-duct lobular units (TDLU) containing CIS are sometimes pierced or injured, so that neoplastic cells may artifactually enter the stroma surrounding the TDLU. In this situation, distinguishing traumatic disruption from true invasion may be difficult. The evidence of *recent trauma* is usually readily apparent, due to hemorrhage and early fibroblastic proliferation in the area of the wound (Figs. 21.1–21.5). From low-power observation, the pathologist can identify the needle track (Fig. 21.1) and compare the cellular alterations within the track with those in adjacent portions of the duct which have not been injured. Carcinoma cells which have been dislodged in such a fashion commonly appear distorted, as either single cells or small groups, and may appear either mixed with or trapped within young, proliferating connective tissue and mixed with varying numbers of inflammatory cells. The presence of macrophages containing hemosiderin pigment may be very helpful, particularly when they are found close to the dislodged cells.

In contrast, the presence of *carcinoma cells* which appear to actively infiltrate stroma around the duct and demonstrate varying degrees of tubule formation or distinct linear infiltration is suggestive of true stromal invasion. The presence of desmoplastic tissue not mixed with hemosiderin-laden cells is helpful in making the diagnosis. The pathologist must be careful to ascertain that these infiltrating structures do not include myoepithelial cells, lest ductules of distorted adenosis or of distorted DCIS be misinterpreted as infiltrating carcinoma (Figs. 21.3, 21.4, 21.6).

In cases of cell displacement related to guide wire trauma, there is generally no stromal reaction such as granulation tissue formation, fibroblastic proliferation, or organizing hematoma in the sample. Tissue disruption in this type of trauma usually results in minor hemorrhage, with displacement of fat cells or clusters of dislodged tumor cells with jagged edges.

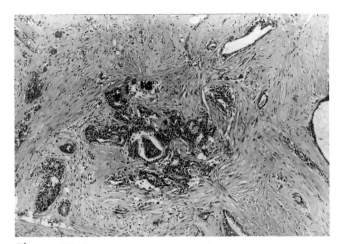

Figure 21.1. Posttraumatic pseudoinvasion.

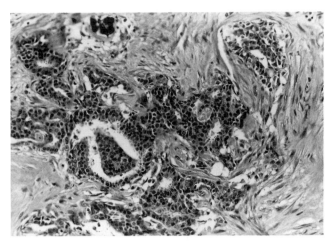

Figure 21.2. Posttraumatic pseudoinvasion.

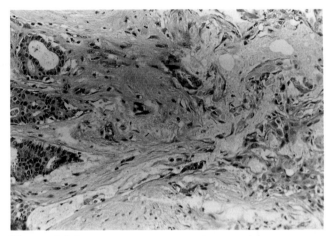

Figure 21.3. Posttraumatic pseudoinvasion.

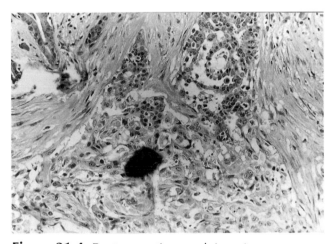

Figure 21.4. Posttraumatic pseudoinvasion.

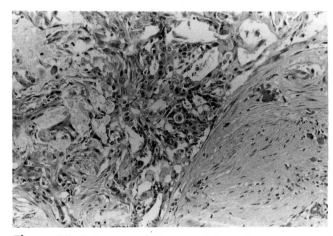

Figure 21.5. Posttraumatic pseudoinvasion.

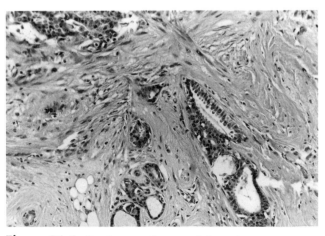

Figure 21.6. Posttraumatic pseudoinvasion.

Section 4

PAPILLARY LESIONS

GENERAL CONSIDERATIONS

Papillary lesions of the breast include *large duct papillomas, multiple papillomas arising in smaller ducts* (papillomatosis), and *non-infiltrating papillary carcinomas* (papillary DCIS) which may be central (solitary) or *peripheral* (multifocal). Infiltrating forms of papillary carcinoma, which are rather rare, will also be commented on briefly in this section.

The term *papilloma* has been used rather loosely. This term should be restricted to lesions with arborizing stalks of fibrovascular tissue enveloped by two types of cells (epithelial and myoepithelial). Ductal hyperplasias of the fenestrated type (usual hyperplasia) which are not supported by a fibrovascular stroma but which may be seen in association with multiple small duct papillomas do not qualify for the term papilloma and should not be designated as papillomatosis (see also Section 2). Similarly, the micropapillary variant of intraductal carcinoma, in which a uniform cell population similar to that seen in the cribriform variant of DCIS forms small tufts and micropapillae not supported by fibrovascular stalks, should be excluded from the category of true *papillary carcinomas.*

Juvenile papillomatosis (Swiss cheese disease) should also be excluded from this group. Microscopically, this mammary lesion consists of ductal epithelial hyperplasia (usually without discrete fibrovascular cores) accompanied by numerous cysts and other benign proliferative changes. This lesion is discussed in Section 5.

Florid papillomatosis of the nipple (subareolar duct papillomatosis, adenoma of the nipple, papillary adenoma, nipple duct adenoma) is another lesion that is usually included in the category of papillary and related lesions of the breast. As the multiple names indicate, however, this lesion demonstrates overlapping histologic appearances of papilloma, usual hyperplasia, and adenosis and may be associated with papillomas in adjacent ducts. This lesion will be discussed in Section 6.

Conversely, a lesion which should properly be included in the category of papillary lesions is the so-called *ductal adenoma*. This lesion, composed of two cell types (epithelial and myoepithelial), probably represents a sclerosed stage of duct papilloma and will be included in Chapter 23 in this section.

A variety of secondary alterations such as metaplasia (apocrine and squamous) can occur in papillomas, as well as infarction and sclerosis. Some of these alterations, especially if associated with scarring and reactive changes, can trap and distort the residual cellular elements of papillomas, creating diagnostic difficulties. Ductal epithelial hyperplasia of the usual type and ADH, as well as DCIS, may be associated with or arise within true papillary lesions of the breast. ALH and LCIS may also colonize or involve preexisting papillary lesions. The involvement of trapped ductules within the sclerotic variants of papillary lesions by an in situ neoplasm may mimic an invasive neoplasm and further complicate the diagnosis.

Papillary lesions of the breast, especially those with atypical and sclerotic alterations, represent some of the most difficult differential diagnostic problems in breast pathology. These will be discussed in the following chapters.

CLINICAL

Papillomas of the large ducts are most frequently seen in the fifth and sixth decades. They are usually solitary and rarely bilateral. They may occur in the male as well as the female breast. They usually present with a serous or serosanguineous nipple discharge (over 70% of the cases). Rarely, a palpable mass located in the subareolar area may be present. Occasionally, these lesions occur in a more peripheral location. Sometimes they are located in a cystically dilated duct (intracystic papilloma). It is generally believed that solitary duct papillomas are not associated with a significant risk of subsequent invasive carcinoma in the remainder of the breast. Discrepancies in reported series exist, however, which may be related to the presence of other proliferative and atypical lesions elsewhere in the breast.

Multiple papillomas of the peripheral duct system are seen in patients approximately a decade younger than those who have solitary papillomas. These lesions are usually associated with background fibrocystic changes. They may present as palpable masses in the periphery of the breast. More commonly, however, they are incidental microscopic lesions found when biopsies are performed for other reasons. Multiple duct papillomas are more often associated with concurrent or subsequent carcinoma. An associated in situ or invasive carcinoma has been reported in approximately 25% of the cases. Usual and atypical ductal epithelial hyperplasia are often seen simultaneously with multiple papillomas.

Sclerosing papillary lesions (complex sclerosing lesions) may be seen in patients with a wide age range (fourth through sixth decades). They may present as isolated masses, but may also be found as microscopic lesions in biopsies done for abnormalities caused by other alterations of the fibrocystic complex. Sometimes they are detected mammographically, particularly if marked sclerosis and distortion are present or if a spiculated density occurs. Rarely, a nipple discharge is present. If there is significant sclerosis, skin retraction may be seen. These and related lesions were discussed in Section 3.

Ductal adenomas, which also represent sclerosed papillomas, may be centrally or peripherally located. Their age distribution is similar to that of duct papillomas. They usually present as mass lesions clinically, but a nipple discharge may be associated with some central lesions.

Non-infiltrating papillary carcinomas (papillary DCIS) may also be central (solitary) or peripheral (multifocal). They are most common in the fifth and sixth decades but are seen in patients with a wide age range (third through eighth decades). The central (solitary) lesions, which comprise nearly 50% of papillary carcinomas, most frequently present as palpable masses. Not uncommonly, they are "intracystic." Changes in the overlying skin and nipple, in the form of retraction and sometimes ulceration, may be present. Approximately 25% of these patients present with a sanguineous or serosanguineous nipple discharge. The sanguineous discharge occurs more often with papillary carcinoma than with papilloma. Multifocal (peripheral) papillary carcinomas, on the other hand, may not be palpable and frequently are incidental microscopic lesions found when biopsies are performed for other mass lesions or for mammographic alterations. Papillary carcinomas also occur in men. In carcinomas of the male breast, papillary carcinomas comprise a relatively high proportion.

It is important to distinguish central intraductal papillary carcinoma from the peripheral variety since the latter is frequently multifocal and may necessitate a different therapeutic approach. Solitary (central) intraductal papillary carcinomas may be treated conservatively by lumpectomy unless there are associated foci of DCIS or invasive carcinoma in the adjacent tissue. Peripheral intraductal papillary carcinomas, on the other hand, are usually multifocal and require careful evaluation of their extent to select the most appropriate therapy. Patients with noninvasive papillary carcinoma have an excellent prognosis. The prognosis of those with invasive papillary carcinoma is also very favorable even in the presence of axillary node metastases.

Although papillary carcinomas are most frequently noninfiltrating (variants of DCIS), infiltrating forms also occur. These will be referred to only briefly in this section.

IMAGING

Papillary tumors are usually soft, circumscribed lesions which do not image well, particularly within fibrous breast stroma. Solitary papillomas, however, may be demonstrated as intraluminal defects on a galactogram. When calcifications occur in papillary lesions, they are more commonly large and coarse and are not highly suspicious. Secondary scarring, as commonly occurs in the complex sclerosing variants, may produce a suspicious spiculated density or distortion on a mammogram (see Section 3). Papillomas or papillary carcinomas which become large and obstruct ducts may create an "intracystic" papillary lesion. Intracystic papillary tumors may present as mass densities with indistinct margins, with or without calcifications on a mammogram. Ultrasound examination may demonstrate a complex cystic lesion with an irregular wall lined by echogenic tissue.

GROSS

The papillomas arising in lactiferous sinuses and adjacent large ducts are usually solitary. They may involve a single duct or may extend along several lactiferous ducts. They are grossly identified by opening the dilated draining duct. The papillomas are attached to the fibrotic wall of the duct at one or more locations. They are frequently elongated and intermingled with hemorrhagic intraluminal debris. If they enlarge, the ducts become cystically dilated (intracystic papilloma) and the lesions may appear multilobulated. Focally, areas of hemorrhage and fibrosis may be present.

Multiple small duct papillomas are true papillary lesions which arise within the TDLU, often multifocally. They may be grossly visible, but more frequently they are found microscopically when biopsies are done for other reasons.

The sclerosing papillary lesions (complex sclerosing lesions) may arise from papillomas and represent single or multiple duct papillomas with areas of extensive sclerosis and distortion. They vary in size from microscopic to 3–4 cm. Their gross appearance may sometimes mimic that of carcinoma. These lesions were discussed in Section 3.

Ductal adenomas, which also represent sclerosed papillomas, are grossly well-circumscribed lesions.

They appear as whitish-yellow nodular masses varying in size from 0.5 to 4.5 cm.

Noninfiltrating central (solitary) papillary carcinomas are usually located in a cystically dilated duct. When a grossly visible cyst is identifiable the term *intracystic carcinoma* is applied. These lesions are grossly rounded, multilobated, and papillary. They have a broader attachment to the cyst wall than those seen in solitary papilloma. The lesions are soft and friable, and fragmented portions of the papillary neoplasm inter-mingled with old or recent blood clots are frequently visible within the cyst lumen. They are usually 2–3 cm in size.

Grossly, papillary carcinomas with early invasion generally do not appear different from the noninvasive variants. However, if a lesion which is otherwise circumscribed or even encapsulated lacks circumscription in part of the wall and there is associated fibrosis in the surrounding tissue, an invasive component may be suspected.

22. Papilloma vs Non-infiltrating Papillary Carcinoma (papillary DCIS)

Microscopically, solitary duct *papillomas* are attached to the wall of the dilated ducts from which they arise at one or several locations (Figs. 22.1–22.3). Otherwise, the solitary and multiple duct papillomas are similar (Figs. 22.1–22.4). They are made up of broad arborescent fronds of fibrovascular stroma enveloped by two layers of cells (Figs. 22.5–22.10, 22.12). The cells facing the lumen are the epithelial cells, which are columnar or cuboidal in shape. The outer layer consists of myoepithelial cells, which are located between the epithelial cells and the basement membrane (Figs. 22.5–22.10, 22.12). The myoepithelial cells are usually flat to cuboidal and frequently show clear cytoplasm (Fig. 22.8). They may also be spindled (myoid) in appearance (Fig. 22.9). The two-cell-type lining, however, may not be appreciated in all areas of the papilloma; when there is doubt, immunostain for actin may be used to demonstrate the myoepithelial layer (Fig. 22.10). Fusion of adjacent papillary processes may result in the formation of duct-like spaces in certain portions of the lesion (Figs. 22.1, 22.2, 22.6, 22.8). Areas of adenosis may also be present in association with papillomas, often near the base of the lesion. Although cytology is not always reliable in the definitive diagnosis of papillary lesions and excisional biopsy is usually recommended, the features of papilloma may be observed in FNA preparations (Figs. 22.11, 22.12).

Non-infiltrating papillary carcinomas (papillary DCIS) also demonstrate arborizing vascular stalks covered by epithelial cells that may assume a variety of proliferative patterns. The papillae of these lesions may be blunt and sparse or filiform and florid (Figs. 22.13–22.19). The amount of stroma within the supporting stalks varies. In some cases the stalks may be fairly broad, consisting mainly of acellular connective tissue and some vascular spaces. More commonly they are extremely delicate, and focally somewhat inconspicuous. Some of the poorly cohesive neoplastic cells may be detached from the main stalks and form small clusters in the duct lumen. Scattered microcalcifications may be present. The individual cells of papillary carcinoma are usually elongated, closely packed, and arranged perpendicular to the fibrovascular cores (Figs. 22.14–22.18). They are often amphophilic but may occasionally be oxyphilic. The nuclei are characteristically hyperchromatic, regardless of the cytologic grade. The nuclear/cytoplasmic ratio is usually high. The mitotic rate is variable. So-called apocrine snouts may be present in the cells, regardless of their tinctorial characteristics (Figs. 22.14, 22.17). Focal areas of solid, reticular, cribriform, and micropapillary proliferation may also be present, intermingled with the more typical papillae with fronds (Figs. 22.15, 22.16, 22.19).

The most important criterion for the diagnosis of *intraductal papillary carcinoma* and its differentiation from *papilloma* is the absence of a myoepithelial cell layer (Figs. 22.14, 22.17, 22.18). It is, however, possible for an occasional myoepithelial cell to be present in some large intraductal papillary carcinomas, usually confined to less than 10% of the papillary processes of the lesion. When it is difficult to differentiate in situ papillary carcinoma from papilloma, the immunohistochemical stains for actin may be used for demonstration of the presence or absence of myoepithelial cells (Fig. 22.20). In addition, according to Papotti and Tavassoli, in the majority of cases (85%), the epithelial cells of papillary carcinoma show positive immunostaining reactions for carcinoembryonic antigen (CEA) (Fig. 22.21), in contrast to those of papilloma, which demonstrate negative staining.

Careful evaluation of the lesion and the adjacent tissue is mandatory in biopsies showing non-infiltrating papillary carcinoma, since other variants of DCIS as well as infiltrating carcinoma may be found in the specimen beyond the limits of the dominant papillary lesion (Fig. 22.22). These findings will have additional prognostic significance and may alter the treatment. Although for a definitive diagnosis of the papillary lesion excisional biopsy is usually performed, FNA may demonstrate the diagnostic features of papillary carcinoma (Figs. 22.23, 22.24).

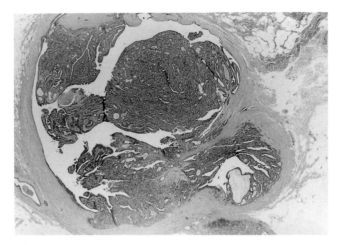

Figure 22.1. Solitary duct papilloma.

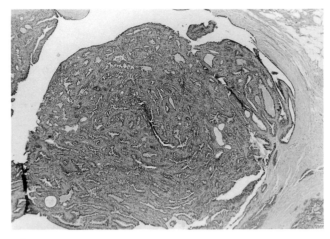

Figure 22.2. Solitary duct papilloma.

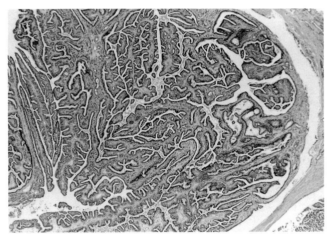

Figure 22.3. Solitary duct papilloma.

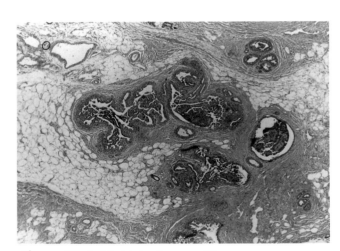

Figure 22.4. Multiple duct papillomas.

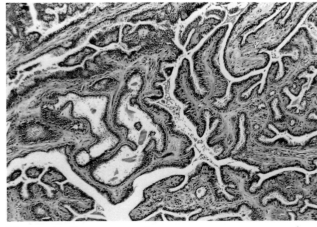

Figure 22.5. Duct papilloma.

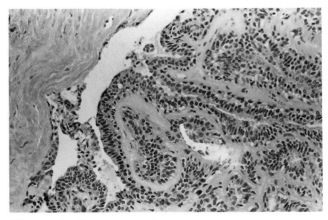

Figure 22.6. Duct papilloma.

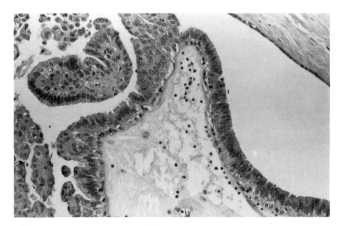

Figure 22.7. Duct papilloma.

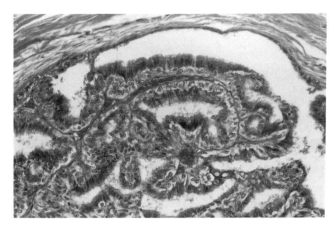

Figure 22.8. Duct papilloma.

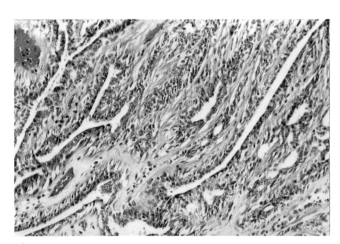

Figure 22.9. Duct papilloma.

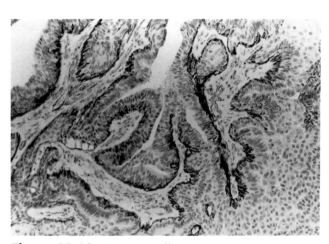

Figure 22.10. Duct papilloma. Actin immunoperoxidase.

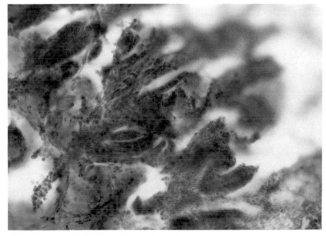

Figure 22.11. Papillary lesion, FNA smear.

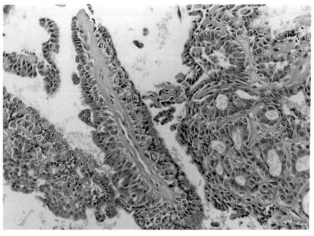

Figure 22.12. Duct papilloma, FNA cell block.

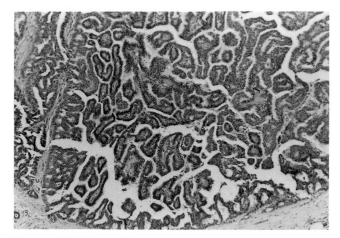

Figure 22.13. Papillary carcinoma, non-infiltrating.

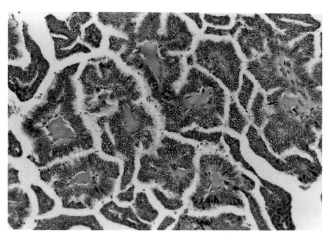

Figure 22.14. Papillary carcinoma.

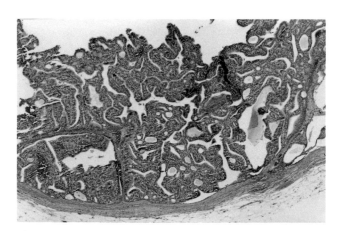

Figure 22.15. Papillary carcinoma, non-infiltrating.

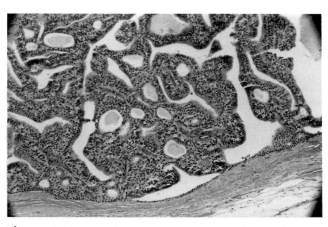

Figure 22.16. Papillary carcinoma, non-infiltrating.

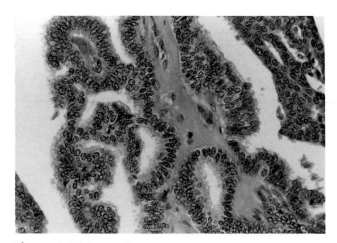

Figure 22.17. Papillary carcinoma.

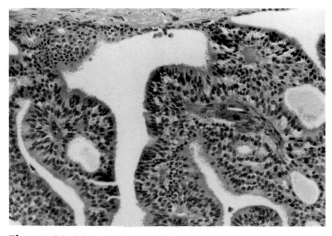

Figure 22.18. Papillary carcinoma.

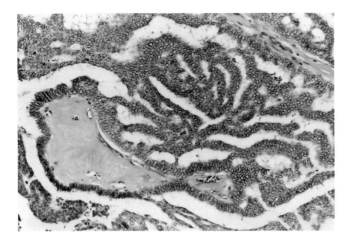

Figure 22.19. Papillary carcinoma.

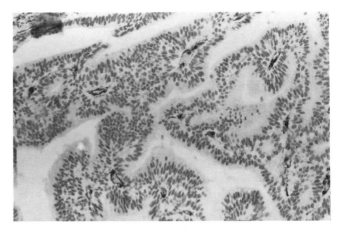

Figure 22.20. Papillary carcinoma. Actin immunoperoxidase.

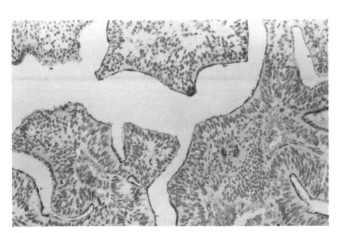

Figure 22.21. Papillary carcinoma. CEA immunoperoxidase, apical staining.

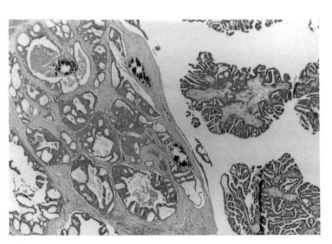

Figure 22.22. Intracystic papillary carcinoma with adjacent ductal carcinoma in situ.

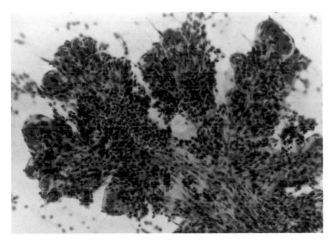

Figure 22.23. Papillary lesion. FNA smear.

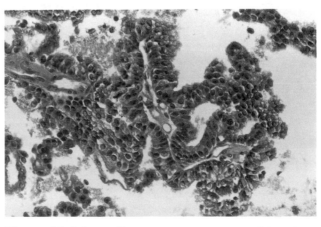

Figure 22.24. Papillary carcinoma. FNA cell block.

23. Papilloma with Sclerotic Alterations vs Infiltrating Ductal Carcinoma Associated with Papilloma

Focal or diffuse *sclerotic alterations* are not uncommon in *papillomas.* Fibrosis often starts at the base of the papilloma but may involve the majority of the lesion (Figs. 23.1, 23.2). Sometimes the fibrosis may create a radial scar-like pattern (Fig. 23.3). Occasionally, the papilloma may be largely obliterated by extensive fibrosis. This may create a nodular fibrotic lesion with rare trapped epithelial elements or a relatively solid but fenestrated and sclerosed process within the thick-walled duct lumen with little residual papillary component *(ductal adenoma)* (Fig. 23.4). The distorted, trapped epithelial elements associated with sclerosed papillomas may create concern, as they may imitate an *infiltrating ductal carcinoma.* At low magnification the papillary nature of the lesion is readily apparent, however (Figs. 23.1–23.3), and at high magnification the persistence of myoepithelial cells (although attenuated) is observed (Fig. 23.5). The presence of myoepithelial cells in residual papillary processes and in the trapped glandular structures in sclerotic areas is a strong assurance of benignity. Immunostains for actin may also be performed to further document the presence of myoepithelial cells (Fig. 23.6).

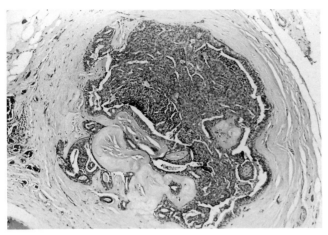

Figure 23.1. Papilloma with sclerosis.

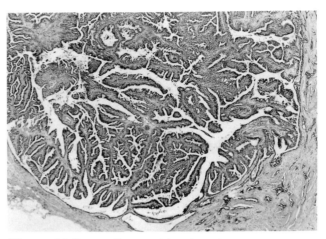

Figure 23.2. Papilloma with sclerosis.

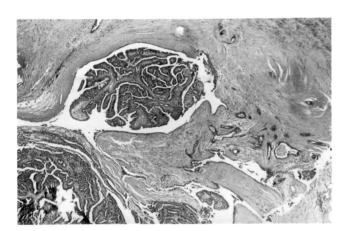

Figure 23.3. Papilloma with sclerosis.

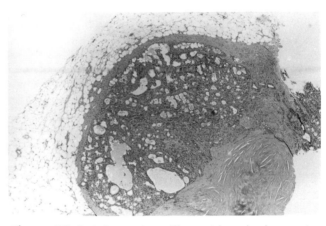

Figure 23.4. Sclerosed papilloma (ductal adenoma).

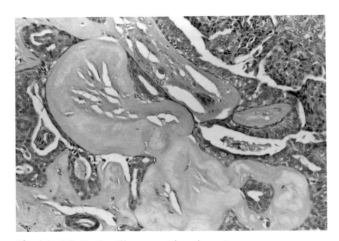

Figure 23.5. Papilloma with sclerosis.

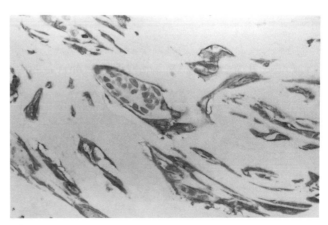

Figure 23.6. Papilloma with sclerosis. Actin immunoperoxidase.

24. Papilloma with Metaplastic Alterations vs Carcinoma

Focal apocrine metaplasia is not uncommon in papilloma (Fig. 24.1). The metaplastic component may also be demonstrated in FNA preparations (Figs. 24.2, 24.3). Extensive metaplasia with almost complete replacement of the epithelial cell layer also occurs rarely (Fig. 24.4). In some cases, recognition of the myoepithelial cell layer may be difficult. If there are also atypical and/or hyperplastic alterations involving the metaplastic apocrine cells, the latter with formation of bridges and cribriform patterns, exclusion of an *apocrine carcinoma* arising in a papilloma may be more difficult (Figs. 24.4–24.8). Apocrine carcinoma arising in a papilloma (the carcinoma must occupy more than one-third of the cross section of the papillary lesion), however, is rare. Further, according to Tavassoli, these lesions warrant the diagnosis of carcinoma only when there is evidence of stromal or vascular invasion. The papillary non-necrotic type of intraductal apocrine carcinoma is also a rare lesion. It is characterized by complex papillae lined by relatively uniform, atypical apocrine cells forming bridges, arcades, and solid nests. The papillary processes of such lesions are devoid of a myoepithelial cell layer. Difficulties, therefore, may arise in differentiating papillomas with apocrine metaplastic and hyperplastic changes from this rare form of papillary intraductal apocrine carcinoma. When in doubt, imunostains for actin may be performed to demonstrate the myoepithelial cell layer and confirm the benign (metaplastic or hyperplastic) nature of the process. Problems encountered with apocrine metaplastic, hyperplastic, and neoplastic lesions in general were also discussed in Sections 1 and 2. In addition, atypical apocrine metaplasia or hyperplasia involving a papilloma with sclerotic changes may mimic an invasive carcinoma. The presence of residual myoepithelial cells in questionable areas supports the benign nature of the process (Fig. 24.9).

Focal areas of *squamous metaplasia* may be seen in papillomas (Fig. 24.10). Extensive squamous metaplasia, however, may also occur in papillomas following infarction, sometimes replacing the entire lesion (Figs. 24.11, 24.12). However, if there is also scarring with entrapment of the metaplastic squamous epithelial elements, differential diagnosis may be difficult. Postinfarction squamous metaplasia can occasionally be florid and, when associated with significant sclerosis, may assume a pseudoinfiltrative appearance simulating a well-differentiated, invasive *squamous cell carcinoma*. Recognition of the overall pattern and nature of the basic papillary lesion and careful cytologic evaluation of the secondary alterations are helpful in this differential diagnosis.

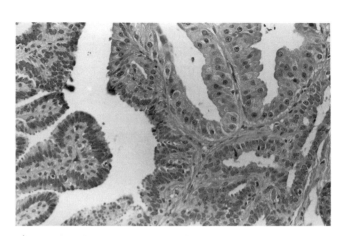

Figure 24.1. Apocrine metaplasia in papilloma.

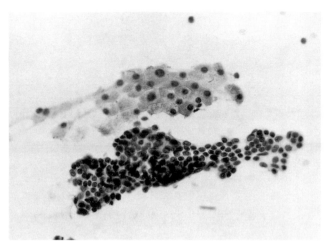

Figure 24.2. Apocrine metaplasia. FNA smear.

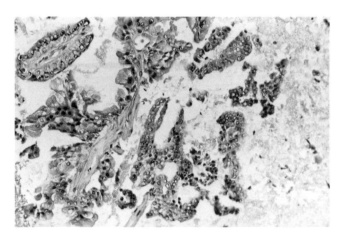

Figure 24.3. Apocrine metaplasia. FNA cell block.

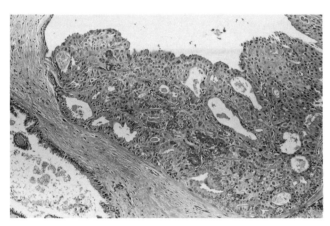

Figure 24.4. Apocrine metaplasia in a papilloma.

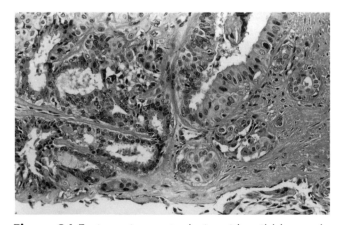

Figure 24.5. Apocrine metaplasia with mild hyperplasia in papilloma.

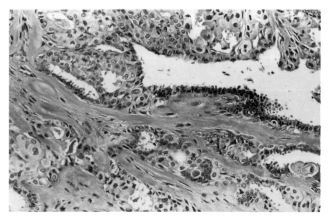

Figure 24.6. Apocrine metaplasia with hyperplasia in a papilloma.

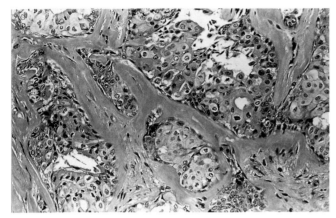

Figure 24.7. Apocrine metaplasia with hyperplasia in a papilloma.

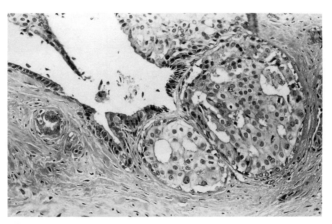

Figure 24.8. Apocrine metaplasia with atypical hyperplasia in a papilloma.

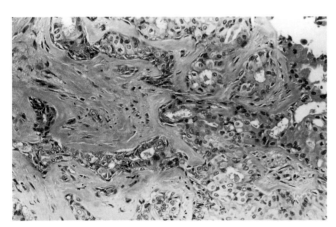

Figure 24.9. Apocrine metaplasia in a sclerosing papilloma.

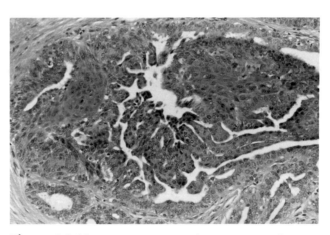

Figure 24.10. Squamous metaplasia in a papilloma.

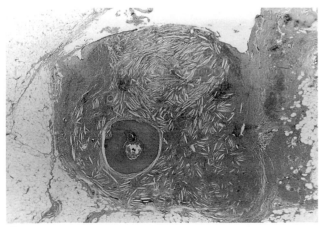

Figure 24.11. Squamous metaplasia in an infarcted papilloma.

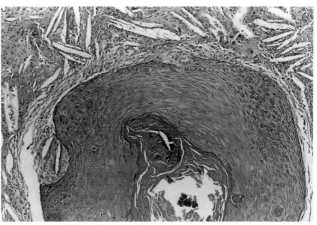

Figure 24.12. Squamous metaplasia in an infarcted papilloma.

25. Atypical Hyperplasia in Papilloma (Atypical Papilloma) vs DCIS Arising in Papilloma

The diagnosis of *non-infiltrating papillary carcinoma* (*papillary DCIS*) *arising in a papilloma* is difficult. The lesions may retain areas of benign papilloma but also show foci of more cellular and atypical proliferation that lead to the diagnosis of carcinoma. In these lesions the carcinomatous component, which is actin negative (myoepithelial cell free) and CEA positive (in 85% of the cases) (see Figs. 22.20, 22.21), is seen in association with portions of the preexisting papilloma, which are actin positive and CEA negative (see Fig. 22.10). Areas identical to the cribriform and other low-grade variants of DCIS which are characterized by a monomorphic cell population may also be present within papillomas.

Tavassoli has proposed that if the area identical to

DCIS involves at least one-third but less than 90% of the papillary lesion, these areas can be interpreted as *carcinoma arising in a papilloma*. If, on the other hand, less than one-third of the lesion shows these *DCIS* changes, the designation of *atypical papilloma* is appropriate. Also included in the category of atypical papilloma are papillary lesions where changes identical to ADH and ALH are present. This may represent colonization of the papilloma by DCIS or LCIS and may sometimes extend along the lining epithelium in a pagetoid fashion (Figs. 25.1–25.3).

The clinical significance of carcinoma arising in a papilloma has not been established, but these lesions may be less aggressive than fully developed papillary carcinomas.

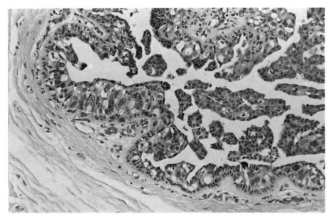

Figure 25.1. Ductal carcinoma in situ extending into a papilloma (atypical papilloma).

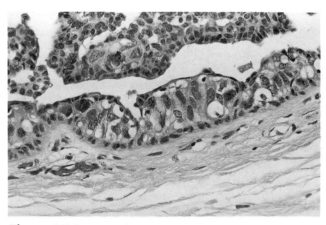

Figure 25.2. Ductal carcinoma in situ extending into a papilloma (atypical papilloma).

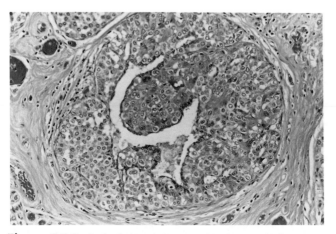

Figure 25.3. Lobular carcinoma in situ extending into a papilloma.

26. Infiltrating Papillary Carcinoma vs Non-infiltrating Papillary Carcinoma with Pseudoinfiltration

A small percentage of *papillary carcinomas* have associated foci of *stromal invasion* (Figs. 26.1, 26.2). The morphology of the infiltrating component varies from tubular to ordinary infiltrating duct carcinoma, and may rarely show a micropapillary pattern.

Not uncommonly, *non-infiltrating papillary* carcinoma is bounded by zones of fibrosis, and papillary as well as glandular epithelial clusters may be trapped in these border areas, *suggesting an infiltrating component* (pseudoinfiltration). This is a difficult differential diagnostic problem but, in most instances, the areas in question represent *trapped epithelium* of a non-infiltrating papillary carcinoma within the area of fibrosis rather than an invasive process (Fig. 26.3). Extension of the tumor beyond the zone of reactive changes, with clear-cut invasion of the mammary stroma and fat, is the most reliable evidence of invasion (Figs. 26.1, 26.2).

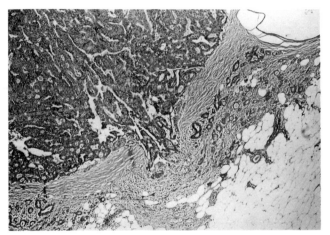

Figure 26.1. Papillary carcinoma with focal stromal infiltration.

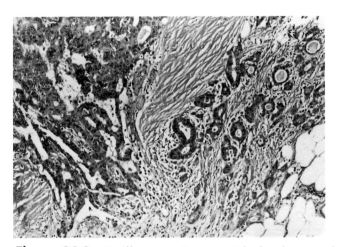

Figure 26.2. Papillary carcinoma with focal stromal infiltration.

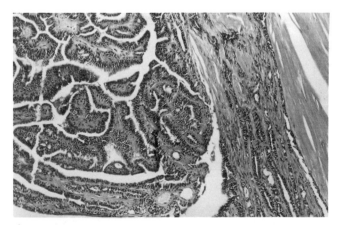

Figure 26.3. Non-infiltrating papillary carcinoma with pseudoinfiltration.

Section 5 SPECIAL TYPES OF INFILTRATING CARCINOMA

GENERAL CONSIDERATIONS

Within the overall classification of infiltrating mammary carcinoma, several subtypes are recognized because they characteristically have a very good prognosis compared to the large group of infiltrating ductal carcinomas of no special type. Infiltrating carcinomas of the *tubular, cribriform, papillary,* and *mucinous (colloid)* types are generally associated with the best prognosis. *Infiltrating lobular carcinoma,* when composed of small cells with uniform rounded nuclei, is also associated with a relatively favorable prognosis.

Medullary carcinoma, while not associated with the same excellent prognosis as the previously named types of carcinoma, is a distinct entity which must be distinguished from other cytologically high-grade tumors (e.g., atypical medullary carcinoma) and must particularly be distinguished from malignant lymphoma in the breast. Other important topics in this section include the distinction between *metaplastic carcinoma* originating from ductal structures of the breast and stromal tumors and metastatic lesions.

CLINICAL

The majority of infiltrating carcinomas are associated with masses. These may be palpable or non-palpable, and the latter are usually identified on imaging studies such as ultrasound or mammography. Occasionally, infiltrating lobular carcinoma may cause a particular problem, in that cases with a paucity of infiltrating carcinoma cells and absent desmoplasia may not produce a detectable density until late in the course.

In clinically evaluating masses in the breast, it is generally recognized that irregular spiculated or lobulated lesions are more suspicious than those densities that have more rounded or oval appearances. All mass lesions which cannot be proven to be cysts or fibroadenomas by imaging studies should be biopsied. Accepted biopsy techniques include fine needle aspiration, large bore needle biopsy, or open surgical biopsy.

GROSS AND IMAGING

Many carcinomas of special type have no particular gross morphologic features that distinguish them from the more common ordinary types of mammary carcinoma. Tubular carcinoma, for example, most commonly presents as a spiculated mass with a prominent desmoplastic stroma, although very small lesions may display only tiny areas of gray-white induration or retraction.

Several of the other special types of carcinoma, however, are characterized by a rounded, expansile mass which clinically or radiologically may mimic common benign round lesions such as cysts, papilloma, and particularly fibroadenoma. The types of ductal carcinoma which are more apt to be round or oval with relatively circumscribed margins include medullary carcinoma, mucinous carcinoma, and papillary carcinoma. Medullary carcinoma may cause particular difficulty on ultrasound examination because areas of necrosis and liquefaction may cause this lesion to appear partially cystic. Fibroadenoma with myxoid stroma may be impossible to distinguish grossly from colloid carcinoma.

There are no characteristic gross features that distinguish infiltrating lobular carcinoma from usual infiltrating ductal carcinoma. Both tumors present most characteristically as a firm mass with irregular margins. Although a desmoplastic fibrous reaction occurs in the majority of invasive breast tumors, this does not always occur in infiltrating lobular carcinoma, and the neoplastic cells may infiltrate stroma very insidiously, so that a mass lesion is not well delineated grossly or radiologically. Breast tissue with this pattern of infiltration may feel only somewhat firm and indurated to the touch, resembling an inflammatory lesion. Neither infiltrating lobular carcinoma nor lobular carcinoma in situ typically produces calcifications, although calcifications may occur coincidentally due to previously formed calcium in lesions of adenosis, ductal hyperplasia, or cysts. Infiltrating ductal carcinoma is more likely to be associated with calcification, particularly when accompanying DCIS is present.

27. Tubular Carcinoma vs Other Types of Infiltrating Ductal Carcinoma

Tubular carcinoma is characterized by infiltrating open, angulated glands lined by one type of cell and commonly by only one layer of cells. Additionally, the neoplastic cells are relatively uniform and low grade, without much mitotic activity (Fig. 27.1). Confusion commonly occurs in distinguishing tubular carcinoma from various types of adenosis and from entrapped ductules in the midst of a radial scar (Fig. 27.2). These differential diagnoses are discussed in Sections 1 and 3. It is important to distinguish tubular carcinoma from other types of infiltrating ductal carcinoma because of its better prognosis and because surgeons are increasingly omitting axillary dissections for pure tubular carcinoma which is less than 1 cm in diameter. Tubular carcinoma is usually suspected at low power as a haphazard proliferation of open glands which may be associated with low-grade DCIS (Figs. 27.3 and 27.4). Closer observation reveals small ductules or tubules which are commonly angulated but which may appear oval or elongated (Fig. 27.5). The tubules have open lumens and are lined by one or sometimes two layers of cells having relatively little nuclear atypia when compared to well-differentiated ductal carcinomas of no special type (NOS) (Figs. 27.6–27.8). Apical snouts are observed in many cases of tubular carcinoma but are not necessary for the diagnosis (Figs. 27.1, 27.5, 27.9, and 27.10). A single crossbar is frequently present, extending across the otherwise open lumen (Figs. 27.11 and 27.12). Occasionally, more complex areas of proliferation may resemble invasive cribriform carcinoma (see Chapter 28), and this is acceptable within the context of tubular carcinoma. One or more foci of low-grade DCIS are commonly seen within tubular carcinoma; this is usually the cribriform type, with low nuclear grade (Fig. 27.3). The pathologist should carefully reevaluate the decision to diagnose tubular carcinoma in the presence of DCIS of high nuclear grade, and the diagnosis should probably be avoided in the presence of classic comedo DCIS.

Several cytologic and histologic features may occur in *well-differentiated gland-forming carcinomas* that are incompatible with a diagnosis of tubular carcinoma. Nuclear features not seen in tubular carcinoma include frequent mitoses, as well as pronounced nuclear anaplasia or nuclear pleomorphism, as are seen in many carcinomas, including rare types such as infiltrating apocrine carcinoma (Figs. 27.13 and 27.14). By contrast, the nuclei in tubular carcinoma usually look remarkably similar within a particular case of tubular carcinoma (Fig. 27.11). On a structural basis, there are limited variations allowed within the basic tubular pattern of infiltration. Acceptable variations include stiff crossbars across the tubular lumen, occasional infiltrating cribriform structures, and portions of tubular wall having a linear pattern of infiltration. By contrast, the presence of greater than 10% of glands having nearly closed spaces or an exaggerated or complex glandular pattern would militate against a diagnosis of tubular carcinoma. It is not unusual to see portions of a tubular carcinoma showing artifactual distortion related to the use of cautery. In general, if a tumor has the overall appearance of a tubular carcinoma and is associated with DCIS with only a low-grade pattern, then focal areas of cautery-induced gland obliteration can be excluded unless there is a strong impression that these areas represent higher-grade infiltrating carcinoma.

The recognition of *tubular carcinoma* as a malignant neoplasm may be difficult in cytologic preparations due to the low grade and uniform nature of the cell population. Importantly, the presence of these uniform cytologic findings, along with the absence of recognizable myoepithelial cells, should suggest tubular carcinoma when evidence of gland formation is present in cytologic preparations (Figs. 27.15 and 27.16). In contrast, the cytology of NOS infiltrating ductal carcinoma demonstrates more characteristic atypical features (Fig. 27.17).

There is no uniform agreement on how much of a tumor must be composed of open tubular glands in order to qualify as tubular carcinoma. The best prognosis is associated with *"pure"* tubular carcinoma, and Tavassoli requires that pure tubular carcinoma be composed of 100% well-formed tubules. Others, however, accept a diagnosis of tubular carcinoma if a tumor is composed of greater than 90% well-formed tubules, providing the portion of the lesion not containing tubules is of low cytologic grade and has low mitotic activity. Carcinomas composed of 75% well-formed tubules may be designated as *mixed tubular carcinoma*. These carcinomas have a better prognosis than the usual ductal carcinoma.

In some tumors, well-differentiated tubular carcinoma is seen in association with low-nuclear-grade infiltrating lobular carcinoma *(tubulolobular carcinoma)* (Fig. 27.18). Such tumors are also associated with an excellent prognosis.

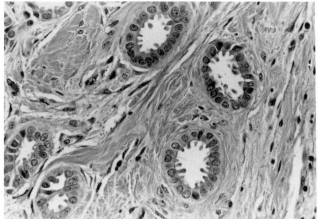

Figure 27.1. Tubular carcinoma.

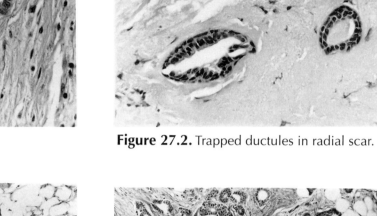

Figure 27.2. Trapped ductules in radial scar.

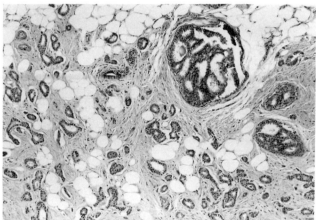

Figure 27.3. Tubular carcinoma with ductal carcinoma in situ.

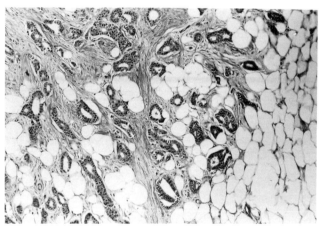

Figure 27.4. Tubular carcinoma.

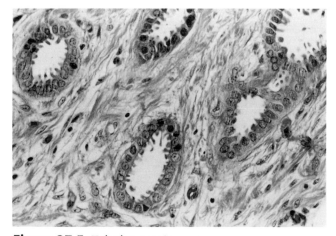

Figure 27.5. Tubular carcinoma.

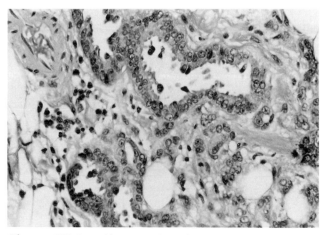

Figure 27.6. Infiltrating ductal carcinoma. (Not otherwise specified).

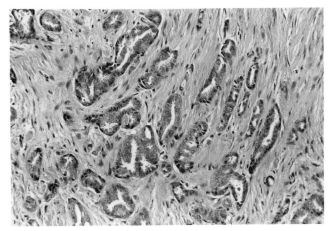

Figure 27.7. Infiltrating ductal carcinoma. (Not otherwise specified).

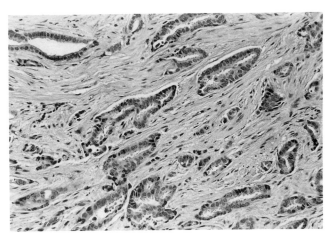

Figure 27.8. Infiltrating ductal carcinoma. (Not otherwise specified).

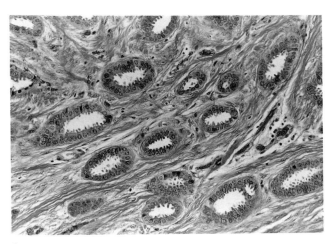

Figure 27.9. Tubular carcinoma.

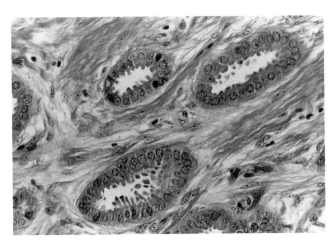

Figure 27.10. Tubular carcinoma.

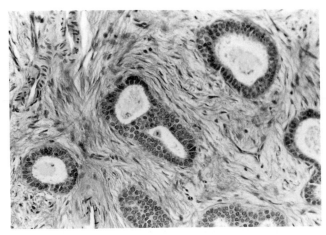

Figure 27.11. Tubular carcinoma.

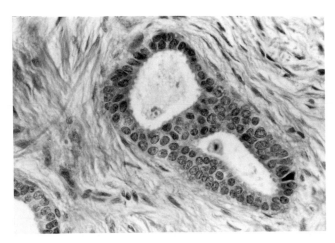

Figure 27.12. Tubular carcinoma.

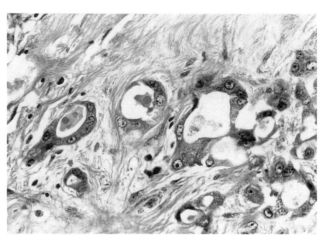

Figure 27.13. Infiltrating ductal carcinoma, apocrine type.

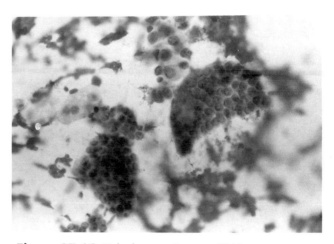

Figure 27.14. Infiltrating ductal carcinoma, apocrine type.

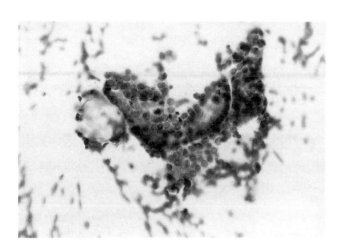

Figure 27.15. Tubular carcinoma. FNA.

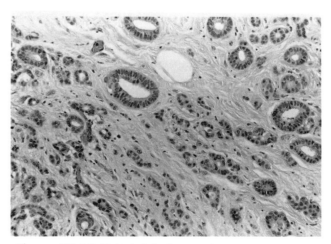

Figure 27.16. Tubular carcinoma. FNA.

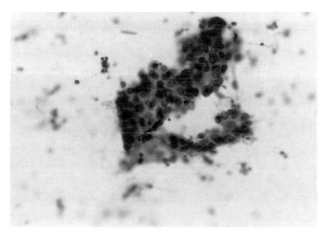

Figure 27.17. Infiltrating ductal carcinoma. FNA.

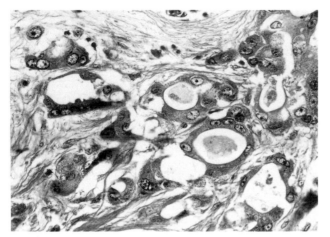

Figure 27.18. Tubulolobular carcinoma.

28. Infiltrating Cribriform Carcinoma vs DCIS of the Cribriform Type vs Adenoid Cystic Carcinoma and Other Types of Infiltrating Carcinoma

Infiltrating cribriform carcinoma is a specific subtype of infiltrating ductal carcinoma which is associated with an excellent prognosis. Infiltrating cribriform carcinoma demonstrates the same low-grade cell type and low mitotic activity that characterize tubular carcinoma, and it is commonly associated with tubular carcinoma in the same infiltrative lesion (Figs. 28.1 and 28.2). Diagnostic difficulty may arise in distinguishing infiltrating cribriform carcinoma from *DCIS of the low-grade cribriform type,* particularly when the in situ lesion is enveloped in and distorted by a scarring process.

Histologically, *infiltrating cribriform carcinoma* is characterized by oval or angulated masses of glands having the same sieve-like internal morphology as cribriform DCIS (Figs. 28.1–28.4). The peripheral components, however, are typically devoid of the myoepithelial layer which characteristically invests all or part of the periphery of low-grade DCIS (Figs. 28.5 and 28.6). The cells composing these infiltrating units are monomorphic, cytologically low grade, and have the same low mitotic activity as tubular carcinoma (Figs. 28.2–28.4).

At low power, infiltrating cribriform carcinoma can be suspected when the cribriform units appear to show haphazard "movement" through the collagenous stroma, as evidenced by a more angular nature of the infiltrative glandular groups compared to DCIS (Figs. 28.1 and 28.2). This infiltrative phenomenon, however, may be mimicked by DCIS lesions which are entrapped within a scar (Figs. 28.5, 28.7, and 28.8). At higher power, the most important distinction rests on the demonstration of myoepithelium (Fig. 28.5) in true cribriform DCIS and its absence in infiltrating cribriform carcinoma. In difficult cases, the demonstration of myoepithelium may become clear with immunohistochemical staining for actin filaments in the myoepithelial cells (Fig. 28.6).

Adenoid cystic carcinoma (ACC) of the breast shares morphologic features with adenoid cystic carcinoma of salivary glands but has a much better prognosis. This rare tumor is characteristically well circumscribed peripherally and may contain grossly visible cysts.

Histologically, ACC is unique among infiltrating ductal carcinomas of the breast in that the tumor is characteristically composed of two different types of cells and because of its special stromal features. At low power the tumor is characterized by infiltrating circumscribed or nesting glandular formations having features similar to those of infiltrating cribriform carcinoma (Figs. 28.9 and 28.10). The punched-out spaces are sometimes filled with a blue mucoid substance in the characteristic "adenoid" areas (Fig. 28.10) or may contain eosinophilic basement membrane material or hyaline bodies (Fig. 28.11) in "cylindromatous" areas. Either of these materials may predominate in different parts of the tumor, but commonly both mucoid accumulation and hyalinized solid material coexist in the same circumscribed nests. Additionally, some spaces are lined by a linear deposit of eosinophilic material coating the lining cells.

The cellular elements are characteristically of two types: (1) a predominant basaloid cell (which may show positive staining with actin) and (2) a larger pink-staining cell which typically will stain positively for keratin. Tavasoli emphasizes that the combination of cell types should be present for a diagnosis of ACC.

In addition to the classic cribriform-like growth pattern, other growth patterns may be seen, including solid, tubular, trabecular (Fig. 28.12), and basaloid. Sebaceous differentiation has been observed in a small percentage of ACC. The cell population in ACC is more pleomorphic than the monomorphic population in infiltrating cribriform carcinoma and in low-grade cribriform DCIS (Figs. 28.13–28.15).

Collagenous spherulosis in association with ductal hyperplasia must be distinguished from the cylindromatous component of ACC. In general, collagenous spherulosis is seen as an incidental microscopic lesion that is not part of a tumor mass or an infiltrative lesion, and the pathologist should forgo any impulse to label these lesions as in situ ACC. Commonly, the stromal spherules of collagenous spherulosis contain internal structures, particularly laminar arrangements or star-shaped, fibrillar patterns which are absent in ACC. Illustrations of collagenous spherulosis are presented in Chapter 17.

Occasionally, infiltrating ductal carcinoma associated with osteoclast-like giant cells may have areas with an infiltrating cribriform pattern (Figs. 28.16–28.18). In these tumors the giant cells are located around the infiltrating epithelial structures and may be seen within the gland spaces themselves. These tumors are usually grossly brown in appearance due to their prominent vascularity and extravasation of red blood cells and hemosiderin deposition. Although some of these tumors have a predominantly tubular or cribriform pattern of infiltration, most carcinomas associated with osteoclast-like giant cells are only moderately or poorly differentiated.

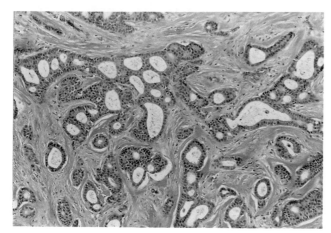

Figure 28.1. Infiltrating cribriform carcinoma.

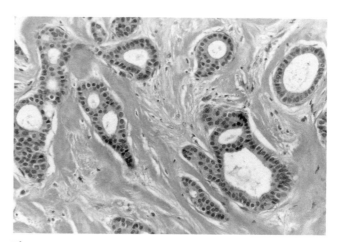

Figure 28.2. Infiltrating cribriform carcinoma.

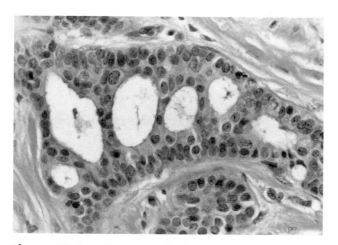

Figure 28.3. Infiltrating cribriform carcinoma.

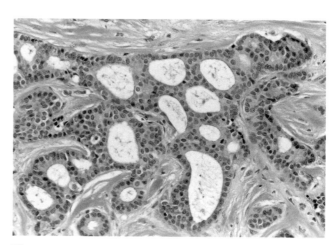

Figure 28.4. Infiltrating cribriform carcinoma.

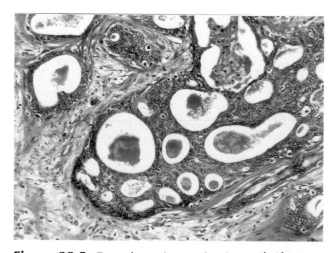

Figure 28.5. Ductal carcinoma in situ, cribriform pattern.

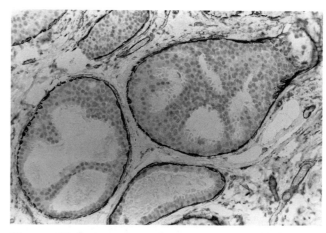

Figure 28.6. Ductal carcinoma in situ, cribriform pattern. Actin immunoperoxidase.

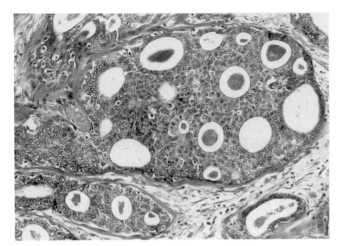

Figure 28.7. Ductal carcinoma in situ, cribriform pattern.

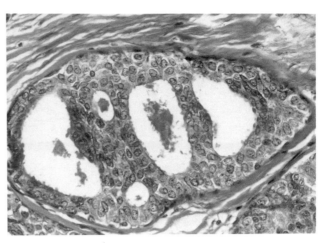

Figure 28.8. Ductal carcinoma in situ, cribriform pattern, within scar.

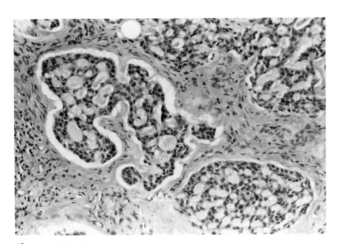

Figure 28.9. Adenoid cystic carcinoma.

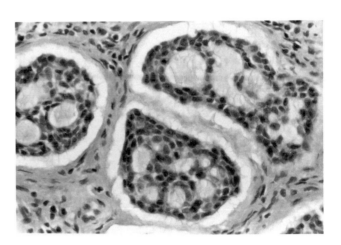

Figure 28.10. Adenoid cystic carcinoma.

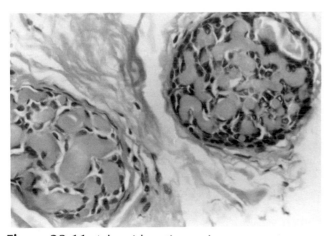

Figure 28.11. Adenoid cystic carcinoma.

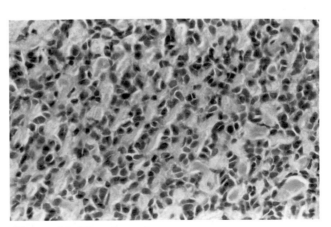

Figure 28.12. Adenoid cystic carcinoma.

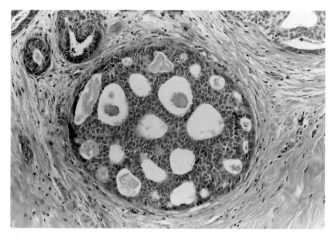

Figure 28.13. Ductal carcinoma in situ, cribriform pattern.

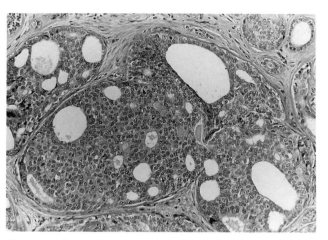

Figure 28.14. Ductal carcinoma in situ, cribriform pattern.

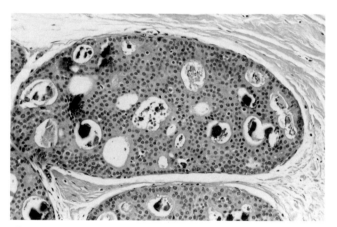

Figure 28.15. Ductal carcinoma in situ, cribriform pattern.

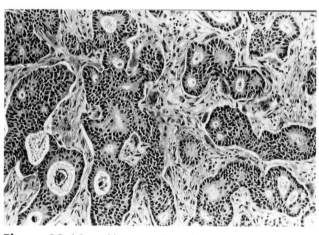

Figure 28.16. Infiltrating ductal carcinoma with stromal giant cells.

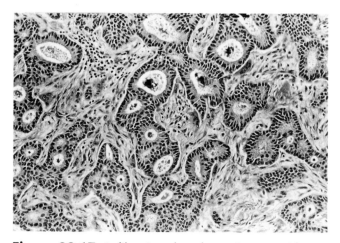

Figure 28.17. Infiltrating ductal carcinoma with stromal giant cells.

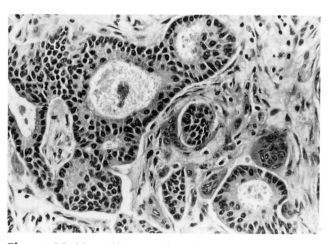

Figure 28.18. Infiltrating ductal carcinoma with stromal giant cells.

29. Medullary Carcinoma vs Atypical Medullary Carcinoma vs Malignant Lymphoma

Medullary carcinoma is a specific subtype of infiltrating ductal carcinoma which has characteristic gross and microscopic appearances and which is associated with a better prognosis than the ordinary types of infiltrating ductal carcinoma, providing the pathologist employs strict histologic criteria in diagnosing the lesion. Grossly, medullary carcinoma is a spherical mass with sharply defined, circumscribed or bosselated peripheral margins. The carcinoma is soft rather than "scirrhous" and may have internal cysts due to liquefaction of necrotic debris.

Histologically, medullary carcinoma must conform to strict criteria. If a particular lesion demonstrates most of the classic features of medullary carcinoma but has one or two aberrant findings, the lesion may be diagnosed as *atypical medullary carcinoma*. The pathologist should be aware, however, that current data indicate that there is no significant prognostic difference between atypical medullary carcinoma and ordinary ductal carcinoma with high histologic grade. Therefore, the atypical medullary designation appears to be useful primarily in preventing the pathologist from overdiagnosing true medullary carcinoma. Tavasoli recommends that the term *atypical medullary carcinoma* not be used in official reports lest it confuse clinical management.

The following strict criteria required for diagnosis of *medullary carcinoma* apply to growth patterns as well as cytologic features:

1. Peripheral circumscription. The margins of the neoplastic mass should be smooth and rounded, as if the carcinoma cells are gently pushing into the surrounding mammary stroma (Figs. 29.1 and 29.2) rather than infiltrating the breast. The peripheral zones are always associated with numerous lymphocytes and plasma cells (Figs. 29.2 and 29.3).

2. A significant lymphoplasmacytic reaction, both at the periphery of the tumor and within the stroma of the lesion, is required for the diagnosis and should be of at least intermediate intensity (Figs. 29.3–29.5). A paucity of lymphocytes should shift a lesion into the atypical medullary designation (Fig. 29.6). The inflammatory infiltrate within the lesion characteristically occupies the fibrovascular stroma between masses of carcinoma cells and may occasionally form follicles. Outside the periphery of the tumor, similar lymphoplasmacytic aggregates are commonly seen around benign terminal-ductal lobular units and in those TDLUs which have been colonized by DCIS.

3. A *syncytial pattern* of tumor growth must be present in 75% or more of the lesion. This pattern implies that the carcinoma cells are arranged in broad anastomosing nests or sheets of cells rather than in tubules, glandular structures, or papillary formations (Figs. 29.3–29.5 and 29.7). Some pathologists accept a minor component of glandular or tubular growth, providing a 75% syncytial component is maintained. In general, a tubular pattern of tumor growth associated with dense fibrosis should not be accepted.

4. High nuclear grade and frequent mitoses are a characteristic feature of medullary carcinoma. Tumor cells are large, and nuclei are characteristically large and vesicular, with prominent nucleoli (Figs. 29.5 and 29.7). Squamous metaplasia occurs in 10–15% of cases of medullary carcinoma.

5. DCIS is generally not found within the infiltrating component of medullary carcinoma, and the presence of DCIS in mammary stroma at the periphery of a medullary carcinoma is not universally accepted. Rosen and Oberman allow the presence of DCIS at the periphery of the lesion, noting that it is characteristically of the same high cytologic grade as the invasive component. In such instances, the TDLUs involved by in situ carcinoma are infiltrated by lymphocytes, and as these lesions expand they may produce nodularity at the periphery of the lesion. Tavasoli assigns tumors with DCIS to the atypical medullary category.

The breast may become secondarily involved in widespread *malignant lymphoma,* or more rarely may be the primary site of a localized primary lymphoma, possibly originating in an intramammary lymph node. In either case, the lymphoma usually presents as a circumscribed, soft mass which may simulate the appearance of the round, expansile mammary carcinomas, particularly *medullary carcinoma* (Fig. 29.8).

Histologically, the circumscribed mass of lymphoma cells is most commonly of the large cell type (Fig. 29.9) and may be accompanied by a population of benign reactive lymphocytes at the periphery (Fig. 29.10). A lymphoma, therefore, may resemble the mixed population of lymphocytes and high-grade carcinoma cells comprising medullary carcinoma. The greatest risk of misinterpretation occurs where tissues are poorly fixed, and the pathologist should avoid quickly assigning such a lesion with poorly prepared slides to the medullary carcinoma category. Immunohistochemistry may be employed in difficult cases to help categorize the cell population within the tumor.

There are additional morphologic parameters which are not diagnostic in themselves but which aid in recognizing such circumscribed lesions as *malignant lymphoma.* There is a marked tendency for lymphoma to infiltrate the cells lining ductal and lobular structures, producing lymphoepithelial lesions (Figs. 29.11 and 29.12). Although lymphoid infiltrates within epithelium may occur in other lesions, including benign breast masses in diabetes, their presence in association with a neoplastic mass warrants additional study, including use of keratin and leukocyte common antigen (LCA) markers. The identification of lymphoid infiltrates within vessel walls is a finding which also raises the suspicion of lymphoma.

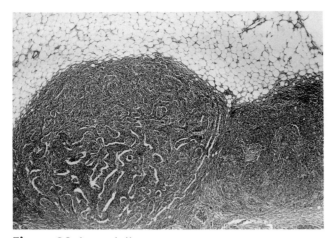

Figure 29.1. Medullary carcinoma.

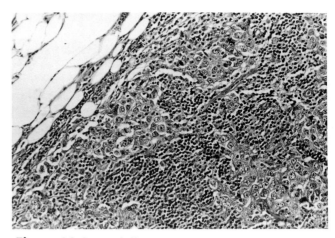

Figure 29.2. Medullary carcinoma.

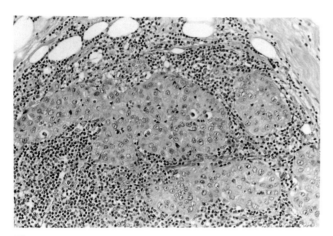

Figure 29.3. Medullary carcinoma.

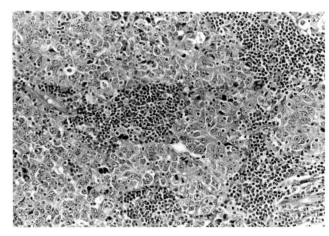

Figure 29.4. Medullary carcinoma.

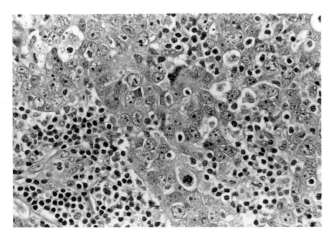

Figure 29.5. Medullary carcinoma.

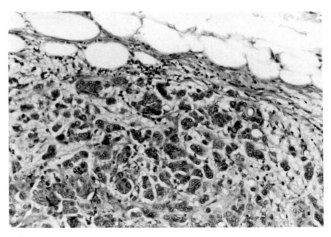

Figure 29.6. Atypical medullary carcinoma.

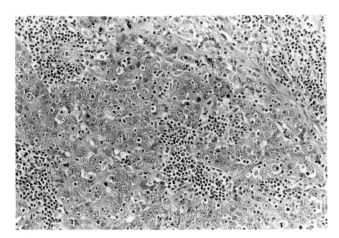

Figure 29.7. Medullary carcinoma.

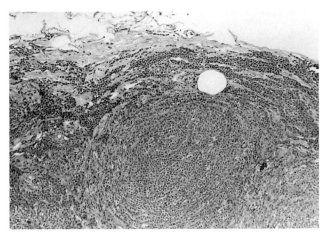

Figure 29.8. Malignant lymphoma.

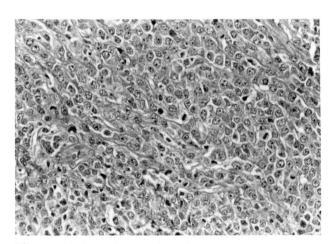

Figure 29.9. Malignant lymphoma.

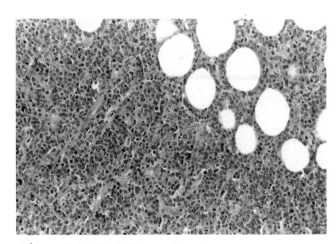

Figure 29.10. Malignant lymphoma.

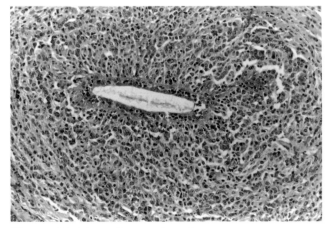

Figure 29.11. Malignant lymphoma.

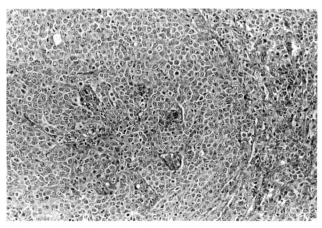

Figure 29.12. Malignant lymphoma.

30. Metaplastic Carcinoma vs Stromal Proliferations and Phyllodes Tumor

The pathologist's understanding of *carcinoma with metaplasia* continues to evolve with ongoing developments in EM and immunohistochemical studies. From a practical standpoint, however, the most important issue is the ability to recognize neoplasms of ductal origin, even when they manifest divergent metaplastic phenotypes, and to distinguish these metaplastic carcinomas from mixed glandular-stromal tumors and from pure *stromal proliferations* such as fibromatosis. Illustrations comparing these stromal entities are presented in Section 7.

In general, infiltrating ductal carcinoma which develops areas of squamous differentiation (most common) (Figs. 30.1 and 30.2), or areas of squamous and spindle cell differentiation (Figs. 30.3–30.5), or apparently pure spindle cell (pseudosarcomatous) differentiation (Fig. 30.6) is categorized as *carcinoma with metaplasia.* The last group in particular must be differentiated from *stromal tumors* and the *phyllodes tumor* (Figs. 30.7 and 30.8).

A second group of tumors included within the category of carcinoma with metaplasia (metaplastic carcinoma) by some authorities consists of those lesions which have been named *matrix-producing carcinoma.* In these tumors there is a direct transition from gland-forming ductal carcinoma to a matrix of cartilaginous and/or osseous stroma (Figs. 30.9 and 30.10). Many matrix-producing carcinomas include areas of mucinous carcinoma. The cells which are apparently secreting matrix in these lesions stain for S-100 protein and vimentin and show variable reactivity for keratin, while the adjacent carcinoma cells stain for keratin, epithelial membrane antigen (EMA), and S-100 protein.

A third group assigned to the metaplastic ductal carcinoma category has been named *low-grade adenosquamous carcinoma.* This tumor is characterized by a neoplastic proliferation of small glandular structures with variable amounts of epidermoid differentiation.

Although focal metaplastic changes in an otherwise usual-appearing infiltrating ductal carcinoma of the breast present no particular diagnostic problems, extensive spindle cell or pseudosarcomatous differentiation may result in an incorrect diagnosis if the pathologist is not careful. Recognizing that pure *stromal proliferations* in the breast are rare, the pathologist should always be prepared to rule out metaplastic carcinoma when extensive stromal proliferations are encountered (see Section 7). Additional numbers of histologic sections are required to examine such specimens adequately.

It is likewise important to identify *phyllodes tumors* correctly and to distinguish them from *metaplastic carcinoma* (Figs. 30.7 and 30.8). Marked stromal overgrowth commonly occurs in high grade phyllodes tumors, and the pathologist must thus search carefully for remnants of the benign epithelial component of such tumors. In particular, the smooth, rounded epithelial contours associated with the lining of the leaf-shaped structures (Fig. 30.8) are particularly helpful in the differentiation of spindle cell metaplastic carcinoma from biphasic tumors, which have a very different biological course and prognosis.

Particular epithelial changes to look for in metaplastic carcinoma include DCIS within or at the periphery of the spindly proliferation, squamous differentiation, and areas of glandular-stromal transformation. These latter areas may be subtle, and keratin stains may be helpful in recognizing gland patterns that merge into stromal tissue (Figs. 30.11 and 30.12). Additionally, the stromal proliferation resulting from metaplastic transformation of the epithelial structures should at least focally stain positively for epithelial markers. Wargotz and others demonstrated that virtually all of their spindle cell carcinomas were immunoreactive for keratin, and most were also immunoreactive for vimentin and actin. Approximately one-half of their cases demonstrated S-100 protein immunoreactivity.

Metaplastic carcinoma and *carcinosarcoma* are not the same entity; this issue is discussed in Chapter 41. Carcinosarcoma in most classifications refers to malignant neoplasms in which carcinomatous and sarcomatous elements can be traced separately to epithelial and mesenchymal origins such as carcinoma arising in cystosarcoma phyllodes. All experts are not in agreement on this issue.

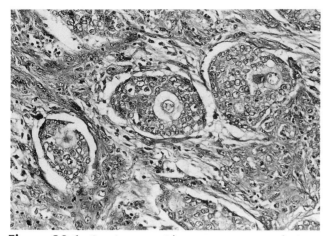

Figure 30.1. Carcinoma with squamous metaplasia.

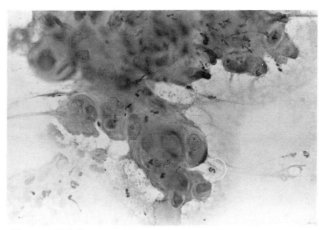

Figure 30.2. Carcinoma with squamous metaplasia. FNA.

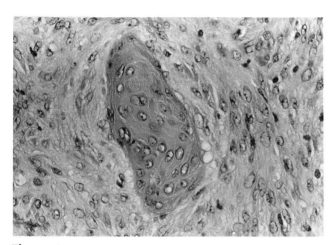

Figure 30.3. Metaplastic carcinoma.

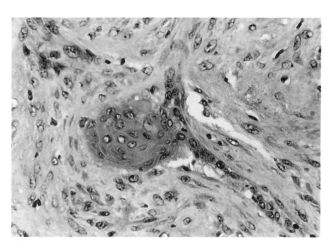

Figure 30.4. Metaplastic carcinoma.

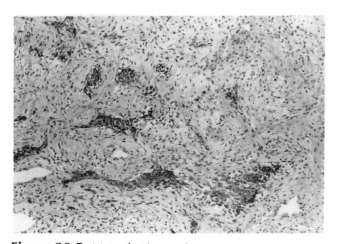

Figure 30.5. Metaplastic carcinoma.

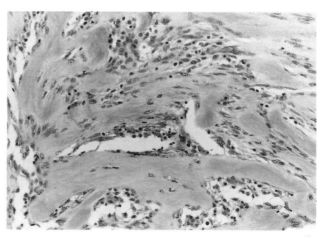

Figure 30.6. Metaplastic carcinoma with angiosarcoma-like areas.

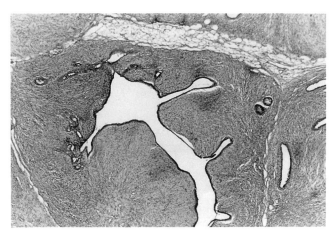

Figure 30.7. Phyllodes tumor.

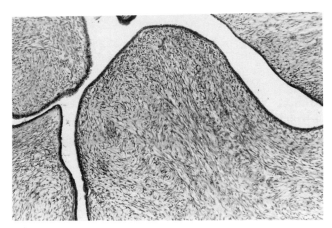

Figure 30.8. Phyllodes tumor.

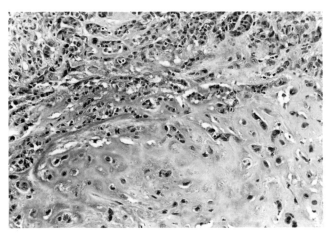

Figure 30.9. Metaplastic carcinoma with cartilaginous matrix.

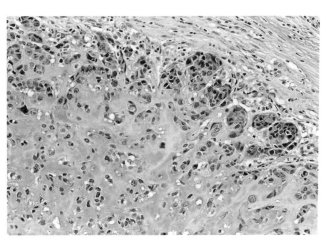

Figure 30.10. Metaplastic carcinoma with cartilaginous matrix.

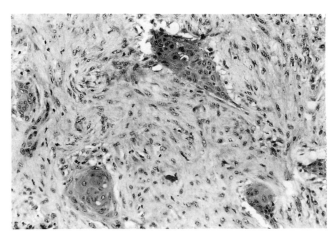

Figure 30.11. Metaplastic carcinoma.

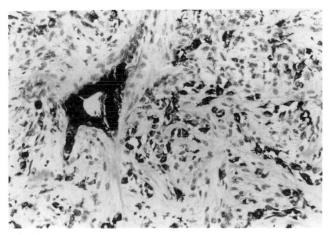

Figure 30.12. Metaplastic carcinoma, cytokeratin immunoperoxidase.

31. Mucinous (Colloid) Carcinoma vs Mucocele-Like Lesions vs Cystic Hypersecretory Carcinoma vs Juvenile Papillomatosis

Mucinous (colloid) carcinoma is a subtype of infiltrating ductal carcinoma that more commonly occurs in older women and is characterized by the presence of floating carcinoma cells within mucinous lakes (Figs. 31.1–31.3). The mucin lakes are in direct contact with the mammary stroma (Figs. 31.3–31.6) and are occupied by a neoplastic cell population of variable cellularity, including some cases in which there are large numbers of cell clusters or solid aggregates. The most common cases have intermediate numbers of cells in papillary formations or oval aggregates (Fig. 31.2). In occasional tumors, the mucin lakes contain only small numbers of cells, and extra sectioning may be required before the neoplastic nature of the lesion is proven. The latter cases must be distinguished from mucocele-like lesions of the breast, where small mucin lakes result from ruptured duct structures.

Mucocele-like lesions are not very common, probably because cystic structures within the breast usually have a fluid or watery consistency, which may become viscid or paste-like but which is usually not mucinous. When the uncommon benign, mucin-producing structures become distended, they appear to rupture into the adjacent stroma, producing small mucin lakes (Figs. 31.7–31.10). These benign mucocele-related lakes are classically acellular, but many actually contain cells or fragments from the lining of the wall of the cyst or duct. The most typical finding is a few cells or strips of cells of both epithelial and myoepithelial types (Fig. 31.10). If the duct structure is lined by hyperplastic epithelia, then the mucocele contents may contain larger groups of cells.

In distinguishing *mucinous carcinoma* from *mucocele-like lesions* having fragments of hyperplastic epithelium, it is always important to look for myoepithelial cells. The recognition of two cell types within a proliferation is the most reliable marker that a cell proliferation is hyperplastic rather than neoplastic. Immunohistochemical staining for actin may be used when the myoepithelial cells are difficult to recognize. Pathologists have been urged to be particularly careful about not overdiagnosing mucinous carcinoma in cytologic preparations, particularly in young women. However, the demonstration of abundant extracellular mucin, three-dimensional cell groups with smooth borders, and uniform nuclei without myoepithelial cells is at least highly suspicious for mucinous carcinoma (Fig. 31.11) and warrants an excisional biopsy of the lesion. Nuclear atypia is often minimal in mucinous carcinoma; therefore, its absence in a needle aspirate or biopsy specimen is not a reason to delay biopsy of the lesion. Small psammoma-like calcifications are often present if the mucinous carcinoma cells have papillary features (Fig. 31.12).

In evaluating slides containing small mucinous lakes, the pathologist should always study the other structures in the vicinity. *Mucocele-like lesions* are characteristically seen in association with dilated cysts or ducts in different stages of distention and disruption but without atypical cellular proliferations. In contrast, mucinous carcinoma is commonly associated with low-grade DCIS lesions of the cribriform, solid or micropapillary type (Figs. 31.1 and 31.3–31.5).

It appears likely that mucocele-like lesions and mucinous carcinoma may represent the two ends of a pathologic spectrum of mucinous lesion in the breast. In examining cases of mucinous carcinoma, intermediate lesions showing features of atypical ductal hyperplasia may be found adjacent to areas with more diagnostic features of micropapillary or cribriform mucin-producing DCIS. In some mucocele-like tumors, therefore, the smaller mucus lakes may reflect ruptured ducts containing atypical hyperplasia or DCIS.

A fluid-filled cystic lesion that must be distinguished from both colloid carcinoma and mucocele is *cystic hypersecretory carcinoma*. In this lesion, the low-power examination reveals numerous cystically dilated ducts filled with a pink-staining secretion resembling thyroid-type colloid (Figs. 31.13 and 31.14). In some of these dilated ducts the epithelium is identical to that associated with DCIS, particularly the micropapillary type (Figs. 31.15 and 31.16). The cystic hypersecretory carcinoma, like other in situ lesions, may or may not be associated with infiltrating ductal carcinoma. This cystic hypersecretory lesion does have a benign hyperplastic counterpart in which similar pink colloid-filled cysts are lined by a nonneoplastic cell population with neither the structural nor cytologic features of intraductal carcinoma. The benign form is designated as *cystic hypersecretory hyperplasia.*

Juvenile papillomatosis is a nonneoplastic disorder sometimes seen in young women that is characterized by intraductal hyperplasia closely associated with multiple cysts (Fig. 31.17). The cysts appear to arise from the lobular units drained by terminal ducts which are filled with epithelial hyperplasia of the usual or ordinary type. The latter consist of a proliferation of epithelial and myoepithelial-type cells without atypical structural or cytologic features (Fig. 31.18).

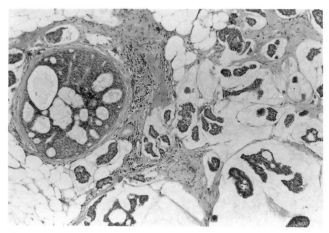

Figure 31.1. Mucinous carcinoma with ductal carcinoma in situ.

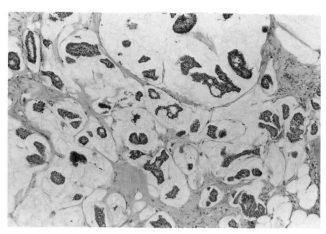

Figure 31.2. Mucinous carcinoma.

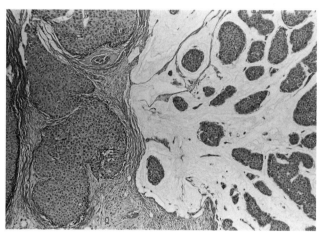

Figure 31.3. Mucinous carcinoma with ductal carcinoma in situ.

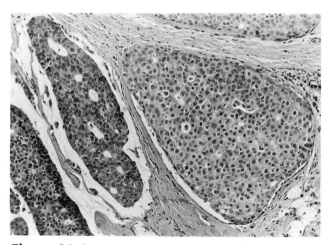

Figure 31.4. Mucinous carcinoma with ductal carcinoma in situ.

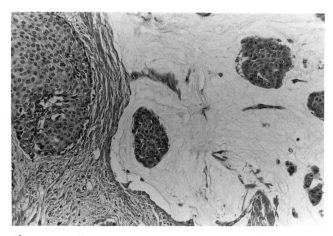

Figure 31.5. Mucinous carcinoma with ductal carcinoma in situ.

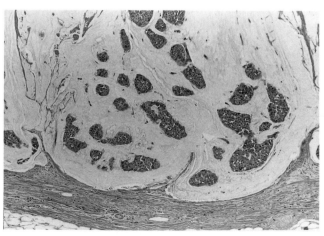

Figure 31.6. Mucinous carcinoma.

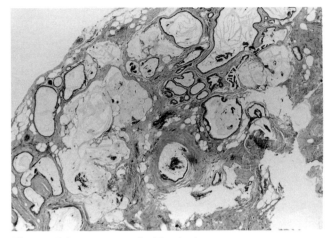

Figure 31.7. Mucocele-like lesion.

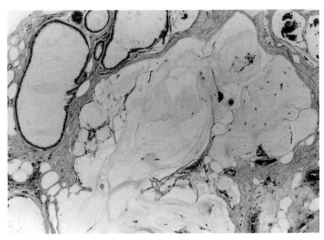

Figure 31.8. Mucocele-like lesion.

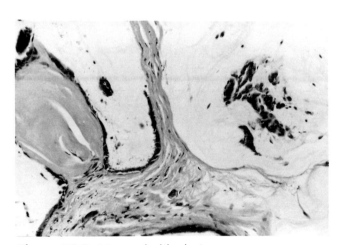

Figure 31.9. Mucocele-like lesion.

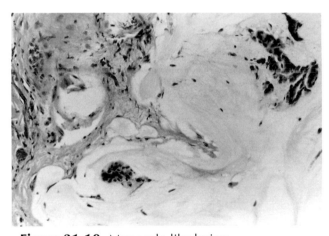

Figure 31.10. Mucocele-like lesion.

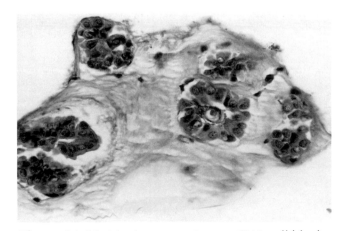

Figure 31.11. Mucinous carcinoma. FNA cell block.

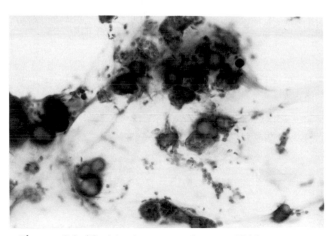

Figure 31.12. Mucinous carcinoma. FNA smear.

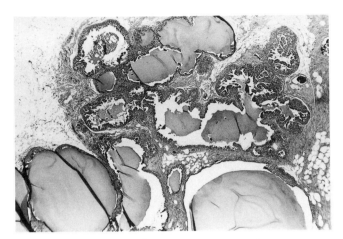

Figure 31.13. Cystic hypersecretory carcinoma.

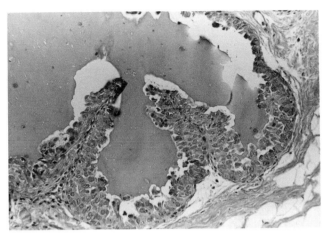

Figure 31.14. Cystic hypersecretory carcinoma.

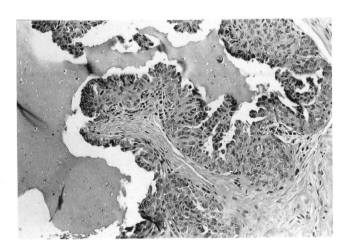

Figure 31.15. Cystic hypersecretory carcinoma.

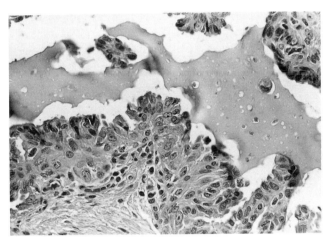

Figure 31.16. Cystic hypersecretory carcinoma.

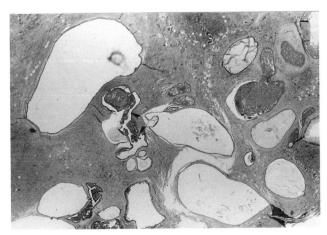

Figure 31.17. Juvenile papillomatosis.

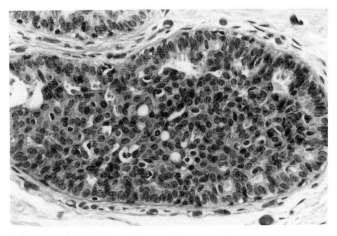

Figure 31.18. Juvenile papillomatosis.

32. Infiltrating Lobular Carcinoma of the Classical Type vs Other Patterns of Infiltrating Lobular Carcinoma

The histologic features of classical lobular carcinoma, particularly when accompanied by LCIS, are well recognized by most pathologists. Recognition of the variant growth patterns of infiltrating lobular carcinoma (ILC) requires their distinction from infiltrating ductal carcinoma and occasionally malignant lymphoma, particularly when confronted by the solid pattern of ILC. The distinction of "pleomorphic" lobular carcinoma from classical ILC is important because the pleomorphic lesion is higher in grade and appears to be biologically more aggressive than the low-grade classical form of ILC.

The *classical pattern of ILC* is characterized by a linear pattern of infiltrating small, uniform cells producing the classic "Indian file" pattern (Figs. 32.1–32.5). On frozen sections, this infiltrating pattern may be difficult at times to distinguish from vascular channels or even inflammatory cells. In this situation, it is helpful to note that in true ILC the nuclei within the slender strands tend to mold one another, leaving concave depressions in the adjacent nucleus, somewhat as if the nuclei had bumped together and left indentations in one another (Figs. 32.2–32.5).

Other features of classical ILC include a tendency for the cords of carcinoma cells to infiltrate concentrically around ducts in a target-like pattern (Fig. 32.6). Areas of LCIS are commonly present adjacent to the infiltrative areas (Figs. 32.7 and 32.8). Cytologically, this classical pattern is characterized by small to medium-sized cells with uniformly staining nuclei and discrete cytoplasmic borders. Evidence of nuclear molding or indentation is commonly present, and at least some of the cells have cytoplasmic lumina which stain positively for mucin. The presence of mucin-positive inclusions is not pathognomonic for ILC, but their presence may often be helpful and usually corresponds to similar intracellular lumina in LCIS (Fig. 32.9). These same features are also apparent in cytologic preparations (Figs. 32.10 and 32.11). When the intracellular mucin secretions are very prominent, they may produce a signet-ring cell morphology.

The mitotic rate in ILC is characteristically low, and this, in combination with the typical small, uniform nuclear size, allows most of these classical tumors to receive an overall histologic grade of I despite the total absence of tubular differentiation. This is helpful in distinguishing the classical grade I lobular carcinomas from the potentially more aggressive pleomorphic lobular tumors with grade II or III nuclei.

Since the time of the original description of classical ILC, several *variant patterns* of ILC have been described which must be recognized and distinguished from ductal carcinoma. These variant forms of ILC are most commonly seen as minor components of classical ILC but may occur as predominant patterns. The variant patterns consist of alveolar, solid, and tubulolobular types. The *alveolar pattern* consists of globular nests of 20 or more cells separated by a small amount of stroma (Figs. 32.12 and 32.13). This pattern is very reminiscent of the histologic appearance of LCIS. However, neither myoepithelium nor basement membrane is present, and the cells of the alveolar variant commonly appear to infiltrate fatty or fibrous stroma of the breast (Fig. 32.12). This pattern has the same cytologic characteristics as classical lobular carcinoma, and the identification of characteristic monomorphic, low-grade cells with distinct cytoplasmic boarders and intracytoplasmic lumina with mucin can usually establish the diagnosis. The presence of adjacent LCIS (with similar cell cytology) or foci of linear infiltration may help establish the diagnosis.

The *solid variant of ILC* consists of variably shaped masses of densely packed cells or even wide trabeculae of characteristic lobular cells (Figs. 32.14 and 32.15). Although conceivably this pattern could be confused with malignant lymphoma or even medullary carcinoma at a distant power, closer inspection should reveal the classical cytologic features of lobular carcinoma with distinct cell borders, low-grade nuclei, and intracytoplasmic lumina. On occasion, processing artifact may cause bubbling of the nuclei and confusion regarding cytologic details, particularly the presence or absence of cytoplasmic lumina. In such cases, slower drying of the slides in the histology lab may reduce this artifact, and mucicarmine or alcian blue stains will nicely demonstrate the vacuoles of mucin.

The third low-grade (grade I) variant pattern of ILC is named the *tubulolobular variant of ILC*. The inclusion of this lesion as a form of lobular carcinoma is not uniformly accepted because of the presence of tubular differentiation. This pattern is characterized by a mixed pattern of linear "Indian file" strands and small tubular structures which resemble small glands of tubular carcinoma, but with some cytologic features more akin to those of lobular carcinoma (see Fig. 27.18).

Pleomorphic lobular carcinoma is a designation used by some pathologists to describe an intermediate or high nuclear grade tumor which has the linear pattern of stromal infiltration characteristic of classical ILC (Figs. 32.16 and 32.17). Such pleomorphic lesions have been associated with more aggressive behavior and should be distinguished from the far more common classical type. These pleomorphic tumors, with linear infiltration and absent duct-like structures, may include mucin-containing cytoplasmic lumina similar to those observed in usual ILC (see Fig 32.9) and may be associated with typical areas of lobular carcinoma in situ (Fig. 32.18).

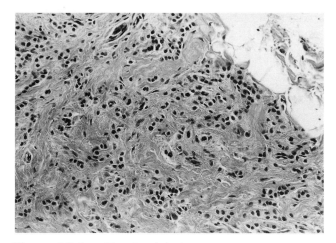

Figure 32.1. Infiltrating lobular carcinoma.

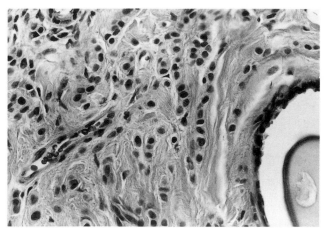

Figure 32.2. Infiltrating lobular carcinoma.

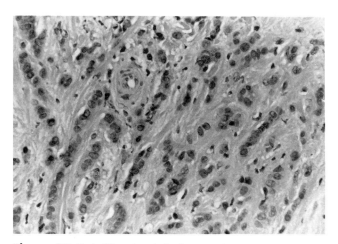

Figure 32.3. Infiltrating lobular carcinoma.

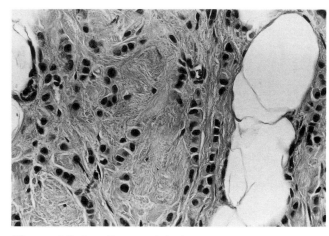

Figure 32.4. Infiltrating lobular carcinoma.

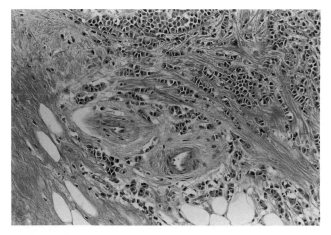

Figure 32.5. Infiltrating lobular carcinoma.

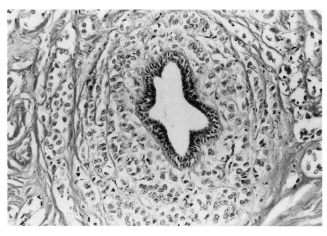

Figure 32.6. Infiltrating lobular carcinoma.

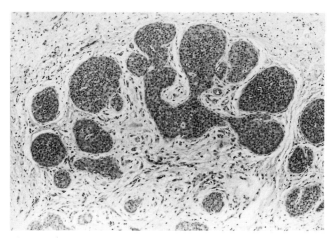

Figure 32.7. Infiltrating lobular carcinoma with lobular carcinoma in situ.

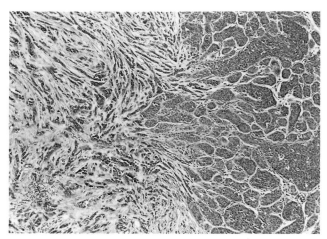

Figure 32.8. Infiltrating lobular carcinoma with lobular carcinoma in situ.

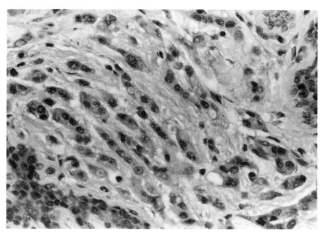

Figure 32.9. Infiltrating lobular carcinoma with mucin vacuoles.

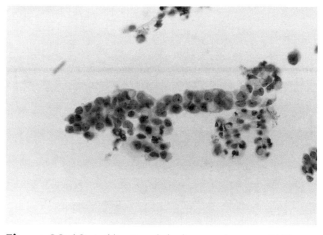

Figure 32.10. Infiltrating lobular carcinoma. FNA.

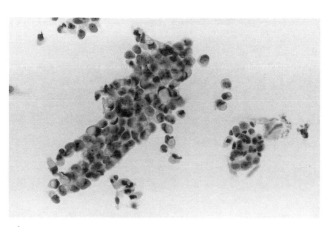

Figure 32.11. Infiltrating lobular carcinoma. FNA.

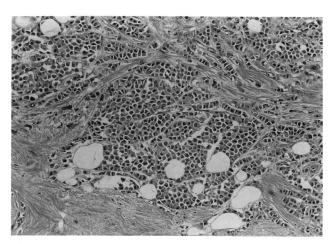

Figure 32.12. Infiltrating lobular carcinoma, alveolar pattern.

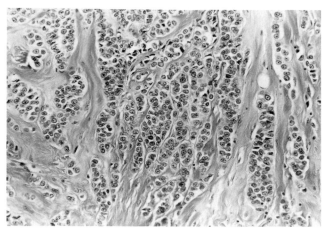

Figure 32.13. Infiltrating lobular carcinoma.

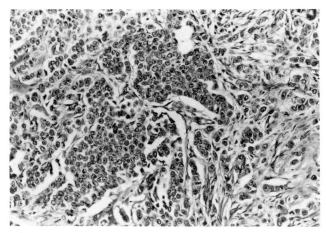

Figure 32.14. Infiltrating lobular carcinoma.

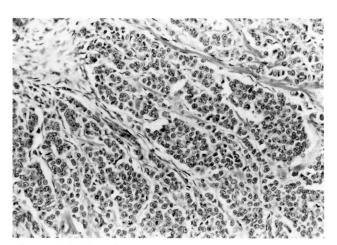

Figure 32.15. Infiltrating lobular carcinoma.

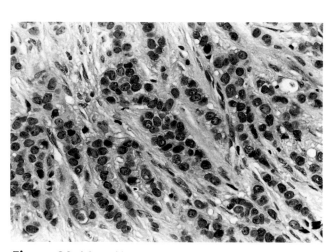

Figure 32.16. Infiltrating lobular carcinoma, pleomorphic nuclei.

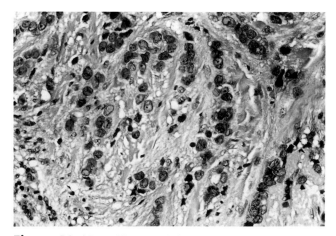

Figure 32.17. Infiltrating lobular carcinoma, pleomorphic nuclei.

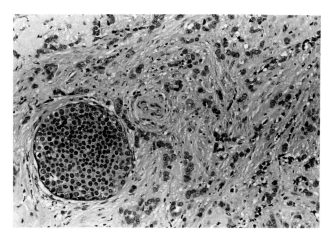

Figure 32.18. Infiltrating lobular carcinoma, pleomorphic nuclei.

Section 6

DISORDERS OF THE NIPPLE

GENERAL CONSIDERATIONS

Neoplastic disorders which involve the nipple may have similar gross appearances and symptoms. Early lesions tend to mimic the scaling and erythema that accompanies inflammatory skin disorders, and physicians are usually advised not to treat unilateral nipple "eczema" with prolonged, unsupervised trials of topical corticosteroids.

The two major neoplastic lesions of the nipple are Paget disease and nipple adenoma. Although their gross appearances are similar, they are histologically very different in appearance, and their differential diagnosis involves other entities. Paget disease is a type of ductal carcinoma in-situ, usually high grade, that follows the lactiferous ducts into the skin covering the nipple. The nipple substance itself is not invaded by carcinoma, and an underlying mass, representing infiltrating ductal carcinoma, may or may not be present in cases of Paget disease. The differential diagnosis, therefore, includes other tumors that infiltrate the skin of the nipple. The uncommon occurrence of malignant melanoma and squamous cell carcinoma are thus discussed in the differential diagnosis.

The nipple adenoma is a hyperplastic and papillary proliferation that involves the substance of the nipple. Its differential diagnosis, therefore, includes both papillary carcinoma of large ducts and low grade DCIS.

CLINICAL

Early Paget disease is characterized by erythema and itching, and may appear scaling and eczematous. As the lesion progresses, there is a moist erosion of the nipple surface which may progress to ulceration. An underlying mass may be palpated or imaged in the underlying breast in those cases where the underlying DCIS lesion has infiltrated the breast tissue.

Nipple adenoma is commonly associated with a nipple discharge which may be bloody and associated with burning or pruritis. The nipple may appear crusted, and as the lesion enlarges the nipple may become swollen and indurated.

33. Nipple Duct Adenoma (Florid Papillomatosis of the Nipple) vs Well-Differentiated Carcinoma vs Syringomatous Adenoma

Although *nipple duct adenoma* may clinically appear similar to Paget disease of the nipple due to scaling or erosion of the surface, histologically the principal differential diagnosis is between benign nipple adenoma and either papillary or tubular carcinoma.

Nipple adenomas appear complex histologically due to their multiple components. In many cases there are elements of ductal papilloma (Figs. 33.1 and 33.2) as well as extensive hyperplasia, generally of the usual or ordinary types (Figs. 33.3. and 33.4), justifying the frequently used term florid papillomatosis. The lesions also characteristically extend outside the lactiferous ducts to ramify within the stroma of the nipple as numerous sclerosed tubules similar to those seen with radial scar formation (Figs. 33.5 and 33.6). While the hyperplastic proliferative changes require differential diagnosis from papillary carcinoma, the proliferating stromal tubules must be distinguished from tubular carcinoma.

Evaluation of a suspected nipple adenoma should be systematic and should involve individual consideration of the different components of the lesion. First, the pathologist should evaluate the noninfiltrative components of the lesion. Papillary components with fibrovascular cores must be distinguished from *papillary carcinoma*. In the benign lesion the cores are lines by two types of cells, epithelial and myoepithelial (Fig. 33.7), as in other benign papillary tumors. Apocrine metaplasia also commonly occurs in papillary areas. By contrast, the fibrovascular cores in papillary carcinoma are lined by one type of cell (Figs. 33.8–33.10), and these cells are usually taller and more closely paced than those lining the benign lesions with two cell types (Fig. 33.7). Squamous-lined cysts are commonly present in the distal portions of the lactiferous ducts in nipple adenoma (Figs. 33.11 and 33.12).

Secondly, the areas of florid hyperplasia must be evaluated to ascertain that they do demonstrate the characteristic features of usual hyperplasia and not those of *atypical hyperplasia or DCIS*. As in other hyperplastic proliferations of this type, it is recognized that occasionally ADH or DCIS may arise within the setting of otherwise usual hyperplasia. The usual hyperplasia within the benign nipple adenoma characteristically demonstrates the pattern of mixed cell types (Fig. 33.13), sometimes with a marked myoepithelial cell proliferation which may be particularly prominent at the periphery of the spaces. Spaces within the hyperplastic proliferation are characteristically narrow rather than punched out, as in the cribriform pattern of DCIS (Fig. 33.14).

After examination of the proliferative areas of the nipple duct adenoma, the pathologist must tackle the infiltrative appearing component. In the nipple adenoma this component may resemble adenosis or a benign radial sclerosing lesion, or both. (Figs. 33.5, 33.6, and 33.15), and apocrine metaplasia may occur (Fig. 33.15). These areas must be distinguished from *well-differentiated ductal carcinoma*, particularly the tubular type (Fig. 33.16). Although the benign tubular components appear infiltrative and do ramify within the stroma of the nipple, they always retain a myoepithelial layer at the periphery (Fig. 33.17), in contrast to *tubular carcinoma*, which consists of a haphazard proliferation of infiltrating glands composed of only one type of cell (Fig. 33.18). Using the above criteria, a diagnosis of nipple duct adenoma can usually be made on core or incisional biopsies, as well as on complete excision (Figs. 33.19 and 33.20).

Syringomatous adenoma is another benign lesion which infiltrates the connective tissue of the nipple. This lesion is composed of cords and strands of duct-like tubular structures which grow haphazardly within the substance of the nipple and underlying breast (Figs. 33.21–33.24). The infiltrating structures are composed of cells demonstrating a monomorphic basaloid appeance with occasional squamous differentiation. Myoepithelial cells may not be identified; however, there is no significant anaplasia or mitotic activity. The tubular structures occasionally produce keratotic cysts (Fig. 33.24).

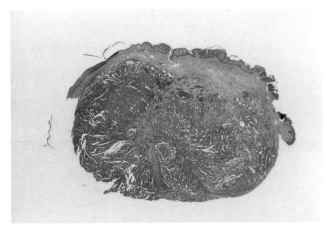

Figure 33.1. Nipple duct adenoma.

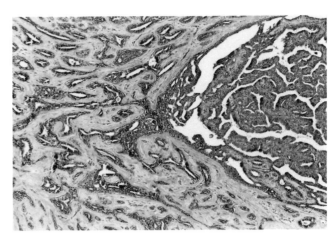

Figure 33.2. Nipple duct adenoma.

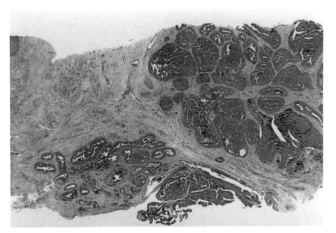

Figure 33.3. Nipple duct adenoma. Core needle biopsy.

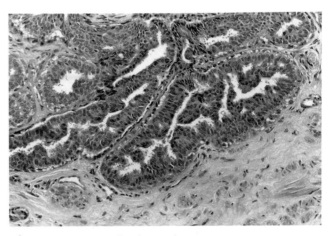

Figure 33.4. Nipple duct adenoma.

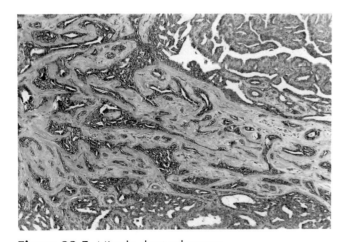

Figure 33.5. Nipple duct adenoma.

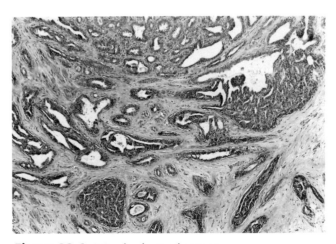

Figure 33.6. Nipple duct adenoma.

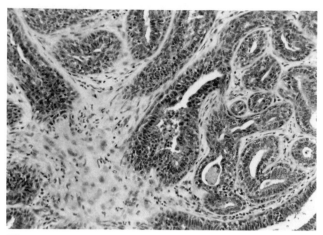

Figure 33.7. Nipple duct adenoma.

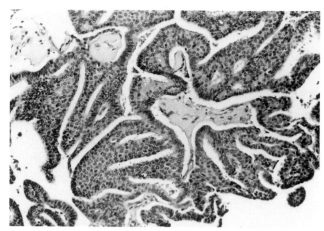

Figure 33.8. Papillary carcinoma.

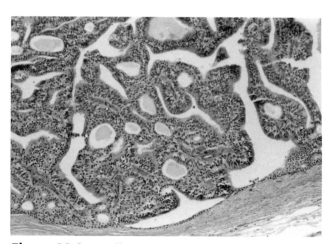

Figure 33.9. Papillary carcinoma.

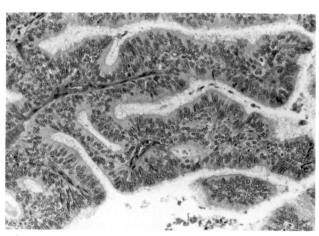

Figure 33.10. Papillary carcinoma.

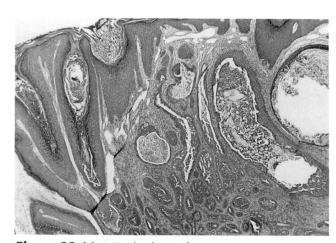

Figure 33.11. Nipple duct adenoma.

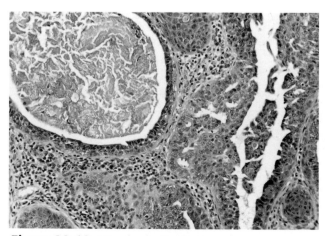

Figure 33.12. Nipple duct adenoma.

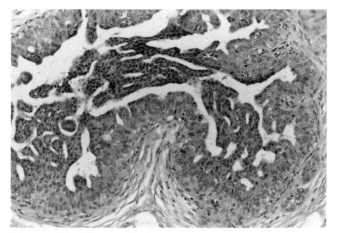

Figure 33.13. Nipple duct adenoma.

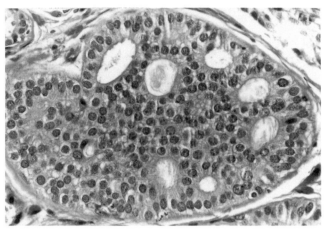

Figure 33.14. Cribriform ductal carcinoma in situ.

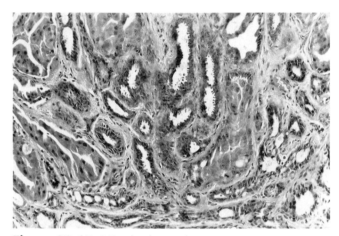

Figure 33.15. Nipple duct adenoma.

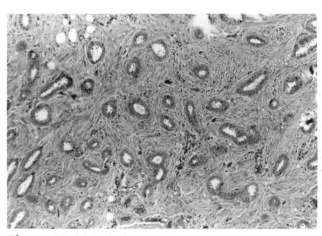

Figure 33.16. Tubular carcinoma.

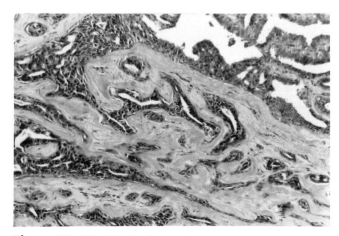

Figure 33.17. Nipple duct adenoma.

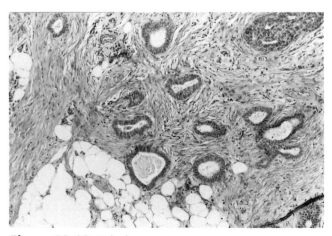

Figure 33.18. Tubular carcinoma.

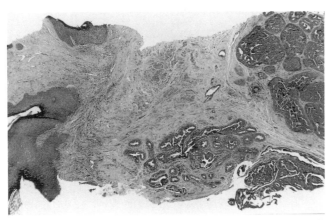

Figure 33.19. Nipple duct adenoma. Core needle biopsy.

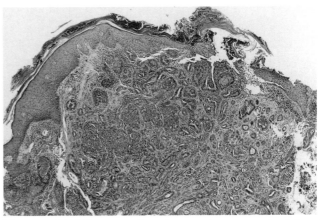

Figure 33.20. Nipple duct adenoma. Incisional biopsy.

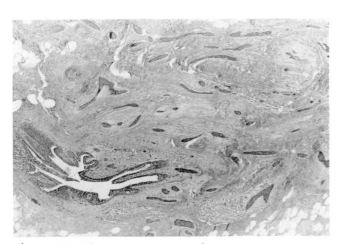

Figure 33.21. Syringomatous adenoma.

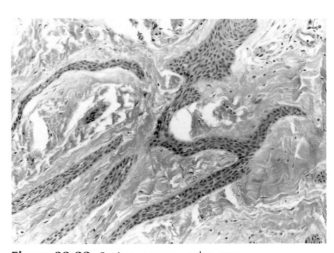

Figure 33.22. Syringomatous adenoma.

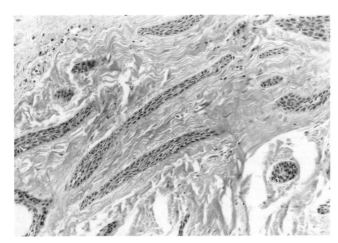

Figure 33.23. Syringomatous adenoma.

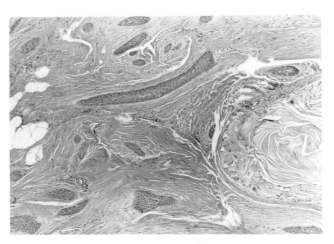

Figure 33.24. Syringomatous adenoma.

34. Paget Disease of the Nipple vs Cutaneous Tumors

Paget disease of the nipple represents spread within the epidermis of carcinoma cells from underlying DCIS. The intraductal lesion may arise in lactiferous ducts just beneath the nipple surface, but more commonly it arises from ducts deeper in the central portion of the breast. As the carcinoma cells ascend through the ducts, they may totally replace the normal lining epithelium of the duct (Fig. 34.1) or may occupy only a portion of the duct wall. Sometimes the carcinoma cells appear to spread within the normal cellular layers of the duct wall by infiltrating between the epithelial and myoepithelial cell layers (Fig. 34.2).

Upon reaching the lower portion of the epidermis, the carcinoma cells commonly appear as clusters of neoplastic cells with clear cytoplasm (Figs. 34.3 and 34.4), reminiscent of the pattern of superficial spreading melanoma (Figs. 34.5 and 34.6). In contrast to melanoma, however, the Paget cells form clusters within the lower epidermis rather then forming confluent junctional nests abutting the papillary dermis. As the Paget cells percolate upward among the keratinocytes of the epidermis, they frequently appear as large single cells with abundant clear cytoplasm and prominent nucleoli (Fig. 34.7). In some cases the cytoplasm of the Paget cells is pigmented, representing melanin pigment transferred from adjacent keratinocytes or melanocytes. The prominent nucleolus and large nucleus characteristically seen in most Paget cells reflect the high nuclear grade of the underlying intraductal carcinoma. The intraductal carcinoma associated with Paget disease usually has a comedo or solid pattern with a high nuclear grade.

In evaluating small nipple biopsy specimens for suspected Paget disease, the task is much easier if a segment or remnant of the underlying lactiferous duct is included in the specimen and that ductal structure contains recognizable DCIS. If underlying duct structures are not present in the biopsy specimen, it may be necessary to utilize special stains or immunohistochemistry to make a definitive diagnosis. On occasion it is necessary to distinguish Paget disease from *superficial spreading melanoma*. Melanin stains are useless in such cases since melanin pigment may be present in both lesions. In some cases Paget cells contain vacuoles of mucin. If this finding can be verified by a conventional mucin stain, then the diagnosis of Paget disease is established. Melanoma is characteristically positive for S-100 protein and negative for keratins and epithelial membrane antigen (EMA). A positive EMA or keratin stain (Figs. 34.8 and 34.9) and a corresponding negative S-100 finding conclusively separate Paget disease of the nipple (Fig. 34.10) from malignant melanoma (Figs. 34.11 and 34.12). Paget cells may also be positive for S-100 protein in occasional cases, so the finding of S-100 positivity does not in itself document the presence of melanoma cells. Immunoreactivity for other substances may also be helpful in documenting Paget disease, particularly the demonstration of estrogen receptors, CEA, and other markers of mammary adenocarcinoma. Reactivity to different antibodies is tabulated in the AFIP fascicle on *Tumors of the Mammary Gland* (1993).

In order to distinguish Paget disease from other nipple abnormalities in biopsy specimens that lack documented DCIS, several factors should be kept in mind. Paget disease is often accompanied by a moderate to marked chronic inflammatory reaction of the underlying dermis, which is commonly associated with vascular dilatation and inflammatory infiltrates within the epidermis. Additionally, the epidermis in Paget disease is often thickened and hyperkeratotic (Figs. 34.13–34.15), and the differential diagnosis of *Bowen disease* (Figs. 34.16–34.18) is commonly considered by the pathologist in such cases. Although this is a reasonable differential based on histologic features, the pathologist should be aware that squamous cell carcinoma of the nipple is distinctly uncommon and that a diagnosis of Bowen disease in this location should be made only with the greatest care. Demonstration of cytoplasmic keratinization is characteristic of some of the atypical cells in Bowen disease (Fig. 34.18), and employment of mucin stains may be helpful. If these stains are negative, then immunohistochemistry may be used. Paget disease stains positively for EMA and low molecular weight keratins but not for high molecular weight keratins. Conversely, primary Bowen disease is positive for both low and high molecular weight keratins and negative for EMA. The stains are summarized in the AFIP fascicle.

Clear, vacuolated-appearing keratinocytes in the epidermis may mimic Paget cells in some instances. In general, they appear fairly innocent cytologically at high power and are characterized by small, sometimes pyknotic nuclei within clear, vacuolated cytoplasm. Significant cytologic atypia is not present.

In some instances, the epidermal appearance of Paget disease is seen in patients with invasive carcinoma of the breast that has grown upward to contact the epidermal covering of the nipple/areolar areas. In these instances, the carcinoma cells may ascend into the epidermis in a vacuolated patterns virtually identical to the usual form of Paget disease.

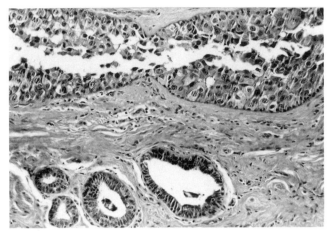

Figure 34.1. Ductal carcinoma in situ in Paget disease.

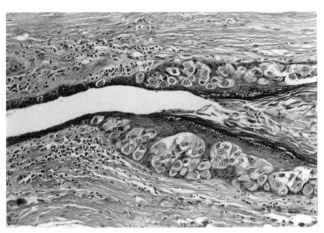

Figure 34.2. Ductal carcinoma in situ in Paget disease.

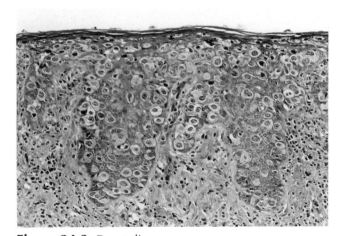

Figure 34.3. Paget disease.

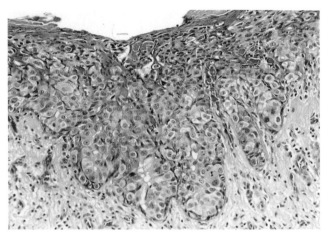

Figure 34.4. Paget disease.

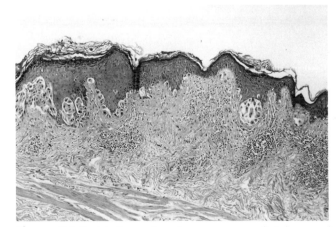

Figure 34.5. Malignant melanoma, superficial spreading type.

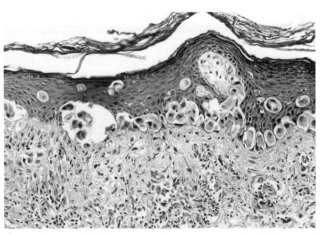

Figure 34.6. Malignant melanoma, superficial spreading type.

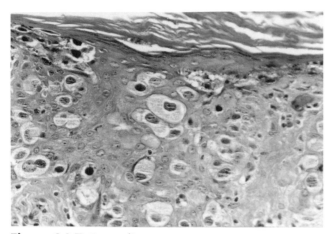

Figure 34.7. Paget disease.

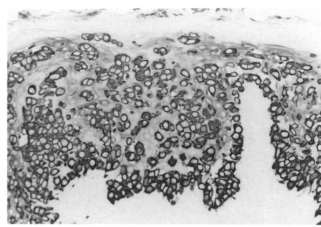

Figure 34.8. Paget disease, EMA immunoperoxidase.

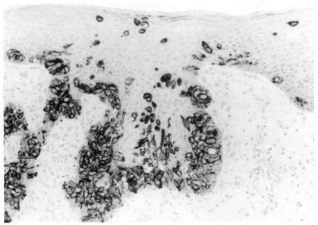

Figure 34.9. Paget disease, low molecular weight cytokeratin immunoperoxidase.

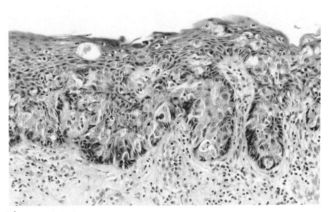

Figure 34.10. Paget disease.

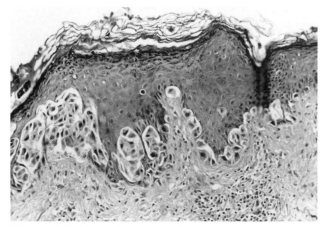

Figure 34.11. Malignant melanoma.

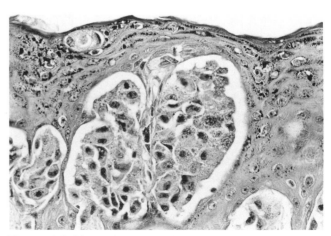

Figure 34.12. Malignant melanoma.

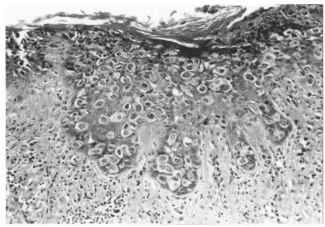

Figure 34.13. Paget disease.

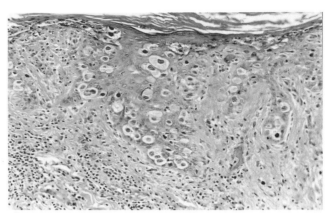

Figure 34.14. Paget disease.

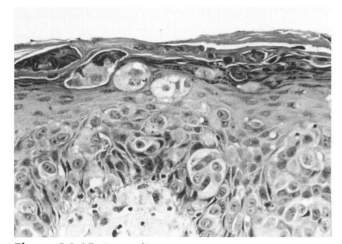

Figure 34.15. Paget disease.

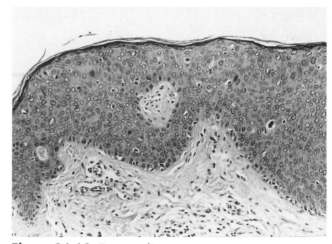

Figure 34.16. Bowen disease.

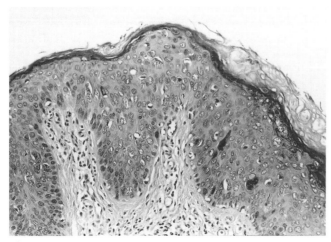

Figure 34.17. Bowen disease.

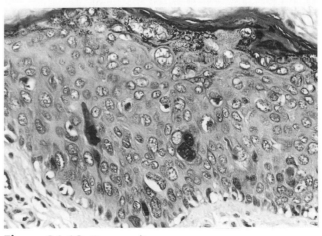

Figure 34.18. Bowen disease.

Section 7

BIPHASIC AND MESENCHYMAL PROLIFERATIONS

GENERAL CONSIDERATIONS

Among the *biphasic (fibroepithelial) proliferations* of the breast, the best-recognized lesions are fibroadenoma and phyllodes tumor (cystosarcoma phyllodes). Juvenile fibroadenoma is a distinctive fibroadenoma variant. "Periductal stromal sarcoma," as recognized by Tavassoli, is a rare biphasic neoplasm which has not been accepted by all pathologists as a distinct entity. Carcinosarcoma is another biphasic tumor that has not been well defined. True carcinosarcomas, however, belong in the category of biphasic tumors of the breast.

Fibroadenoma is a common benign tumor of the breast characterized by proliferation of the epithelial and stromal elements of the terminal ductal-lobular units. *Juvenile fibroadenoma* is a clinically and morphologically distinctive fibroadenoma variant which is most often seen in adolescents. This lesion is characterized by rapid growth and large size and should not be confused with massive fibroadenomas of the adult type, which can also occur in adolescent females. Although the term giant fibroadenoma may be applicable to the large fibroadenomas of the adult type occurring in juveniles (based on the size only), this term should not be used interchangeably with juvenile fibroadenoma and benign phyllodes tumor, as it has often been in the past. The distinction between these lesions rests solely on the microscopic features, independent of size.

Phyllodes tumor is a rather uncommon tumor composed of benign epithelial elements similar to those of fibroadenoma, with a hypercellular spindle cell stroma which is sometimes sarcomatous. The term *cystosarcoma phyllodes* was coined by Mueller in 1838 to describe a fleshy tumor characterized by leaf-like processes growing into cystic spaces. Although Mueller believed that it was benign, clearly malignant forms of the lesion were later documented. Numerous other names have since been proposed for the lesion, including *phyllodes tumor* (WHO, 1981), which has gained significant acceptance. The term *cystosarcoma phyllodes*, however, still continues to be used by many pathologists. The biologic behavior of the phyllodes tumor is difficult to predict, and the histologic classifica-

tion has also been a problem. These features of the lesion will be discussed in detail in Chapter 38.

"Periductal stromal sarcoma" is a term used by Tavassoli for a specific and rare biphasic tumor of the breast characterized by a cellular sarcomatous spindle cell proliferation around open ducts in the absence of a leaf-like (phyllodes) pattern. This lesion, however, has not been widely recognized as a distinct entity, and similar terms (hypercellular periductal stromal tumor, cellular periductal stromal tumor, periductal stromal tumor, and periductal sarcoma) have been used or proposed by others as alternate designations for phyllodes tumor.

Mammary *carcinosarcoma* is rare and has not been well defined. According to Tavassoli, the lesions that may belong in this category include tumors which represent carcinomas arising in high-grade phyllodes tumors, as well as biphasic malignant tumors that have no origin in phyllodes tumor or fibroadenoma and in which the sarcomatous component fails to display positivity for cytokeratin. The subject of carcinosarcoma, however, is rather controversial, and many experts consider most of these malignant biphasic lesions *carcinomas with metaplasia*, except for those with a background of high-grade phyllodes tumor and possibly the rare collision tumors. This subject will be discussed further in Chapter 41.

Mesenchymal proliferations of the breast include a variety of *benign mesenchymal tumors* which may arise from different components of the breast stroma. These lesions are morphologically identical to the soft tissue lesions occurring in other parts of the body. Included in this category are various types of hemangiomas, lipomas, smooth muscle tumors, and nerve sheath tumors including granular cell tumors. Also included in the category of benign mesenchymal proliferations are *fibromatosis*, a locally aggressive tumor-like proliferation which may be confused with malignant neoplasms, and *pseudoangiomatous hyperplasia* of mammary stroma, which is not a vasoformative proliferation but may be mistaken histologically for well-differentiated angiosarcoma.

Primary *sarcomas* of the breast are rare. Many of the soft tissue sarcomas that occur elsewhere in the body may involve the breast tissue. Therefore, the breast sarcomas are categorized histogenetically according to the existing soft tissue classification. The term *stromal sarcoma* was proposed earlier for a pure spindle cell sarcoma of the breast, thought to arise from the specialized breast stroma. These tumors, which are composed of fibroblasts and myofibroblasts, are now classified as spindle cell sarcomas, not otherwise specified. Other sarcomas that may be encountered in the breast include liposarcoma, chondrosarcoma, osteogenic sarcoma, rhabdomyosarcoma, malignant fibrous histiocytoma, and angiosarcoma. All of these lesions except angiosarcoma occur more often as a component of phyllodes tumor or carcinosarcoma, but they may also be seen in pure form.

The differential diagnostic problems encountered with various biphasic and mesenchymal lesions of the breast will be discussed in the following chapters.

CLINICAL

Fibroadenomas are the most common breast tumors in adolescents and women of childbearing age. The average age of the patients is 20–25 years. The lesions present as painless, well-circumscribed, freely movable masses. They are usually solitary, but multiple lesions or successive lesions in one or both breasts may occur in approximately 15–20% of the cases. Fibroadenomas with myxoid stroma are sometimes seen as a component of Carney's complex in association with cardiac and cutaneous myxomas, spotty pigmentation, and endocrine overactivity. Fibroadenomas often reach 2 to 3 cm in diameter, but much larger lesions may occur in adolescence, more frequently in blacks. They are less common in postmenopausal women, and when they occur they are small and sclerotic in appearance. Fibroadenomas are thought to be the result of unopposed estrogenic influence on the susceptible tissue. Some lesions may increase slightly in size during pregnancy, followed by regression after delivery.

Fibroadenomas are believed to constitute a mild but long-term risk factor for subsequent development of carcinoma. More recent studies by Dupont and Page, however, demonstrate that the histologic features of fibroadenoma influence the risk of breast cancer. While the risk of invasive breast cancer is shown by these authors to be 2.17 times higher in patients with fibroadenoma that in controls, an increase in the relative risk has been documented in patients with complex fibroadenomas (those lesions showing superimposed cysts, sclerosing adenosis, epithelial calcifications, and papillary apocrine changes) and in patients with associ-

ated proliferative disease in the adjacent parenchyma (to 3.10 and 3.88 times, respectively). This study has also demonstrated that patients with a family history of breast cancer and complex fibroadenoma had a relative risk of 3.72, compared with controls with a family history. Women with noncomplex fibroadenomas who have neither adjacent proliferative disease nor a family history of breast cancer were found not to have an elevated risk for the development of carcinoma.

Juvenile fibroadenomas most often occur in adolescent females. They grow rapidly and may reach very large proportions. They may be solitary or multiple. These lesions, however, are not restricted to juveniles; histologically similar lesions may also occur in patients older than 20 years of age.

Phyllodes tumor is seen in women with a wide age range. These lesions are most common in the fourth and fifth decades, with an average age of 45 years. They rarely affect children and men. The patients characteristically present with a discrete palpable breast mass, which is usually painless and freely movable. Some tumors may grow rapidly, reaching massive proportions. Others may be associated with onset of rapid growth of a preexisting small mass. Some of the large lesions may show stretching or even ulceration of the overlying skin, but these features do not indicate malignancy. Recurrences develop in approximately one-third of the phyllodes tumors and in one-half of those associated with metastases. Metastases develop in up to 10% of unselected cases and are characteristically hematogenous. Lymph node metastases are uncommon. Direct extension of the tumor to vital structures, with resultant mortality, has also been reported rarely in recurrent tumors. The phyllodes tumors are treated by wide local excision with a margin of uninvolved breast tissue, unless a large tumor size or invasive margins require simple mastectomy for total excision of the lesion.

True carcinosarcomas of the breast are rare. The lesions included in this category usually present as palpable masses. They are seen most commonly in the fifth decade. The tumors may become fixed to the skin or the underlying chest wall. Carcinosarcomas are highly aggressive neoplasms.

Among the *benign mesenchymal proliferations* of the breast, those that may cause differential diagnostic problems include a variety of benign vascular lesions, pseudoangiomatous hyperplasia of mammary stroma, fibromatosis, and, rarely, the granular cell tumors.

Hemangiomas may be microscopic findings or present as palpable lesions. Perilobular and periductal hemangiomas are usually microscopic and incidental findings. Various other histologic types of hemangioma and other benign vascular proliferations also occur in the breast. These lesions are usually larger than 0.5 cm in diameter and palpable.

Pseudoangiomatous hyperplasia of mammary stroma represents an unusual and exaggerated response of the breast stroma to hormonal stimuli. It is usually seen in young women, but it may also occur in older women receiving estrogen replacement therapy. When the lesions present as discrete, painless masses, they are usually firm and rubbery. Microscopic forms of the lesion, however, are more frequent and are often seen in association with a variety of other breast lesions.

Fibromatosis is a locally aggressive lesion. It occurs in many anatomic sites as well as in the abdominal wall, the latter usually in association with pregnancy. Fibromatosis of the breast may be seen in women with a wide age range, most commonly in the third and fourth decades. Rare cases occurring with Gardner's syndrome and in association with breast implants have been reported, as well as a few bilateral cases. Fibromatosis presents as a painless, firm or hard mass in the breast which may mimic carcinoma clinically. Skin dimpling and nipple retraction may also be present. Rarely, the lesions may be detected by mammography. Recurrences develop in approximately 20% of the cases, especially if the lesion is not treated by wide local excision. Multiple recurrences are not uncommon.

Granular cell tumor is another lesion which may present as a mass lesion in the breast, and may sometimes mimic carcinoma clinically as well as mammographically. These lesions are usually seen in the female breast and occur in a wide age range (20–70 years). They are rare in the male breast. Other *benign mesenchymal tumors* of the breast usually present as mass lesions.

Primary *mammary sarcomas* constitute less than 1% of all malignant neoplasms of the breast. They occur in a wide age range but are most commonly seen in the fourth, fifth, and sixth decades. Rare cases also occur in men. The sarcomas of the breast often present as rapidly enlarging masses, usually with no clinically apparent previous abnormality. Breast sarcomas spread by the bloodstream, most frequently to the lungs. The axillary lymph node metastases are extremely rare. When there is lymph node involvement, this often represents contiguous spread of the tumor. Sarcomas of the breast are treated by total excision or simple mastectomy according to the size and the histologic grade. Adjuvant chemotherapy is also used for high-grade sarcomas. The overall prognosis of the breast sarcomas is uncertain. However, high-grade lesions appear to have a prognosis similar to that of comparable sarcomas of the extremities.

The *angiosarcomas of the breast*, which may be seen in younger women (third and fourth decades), usually present as painless and often discrete mass lesions, and they may grow rapidly. Sometimes they present without clinically discrete masses but with diffuse enlargement of the breast. When large, they may be associated with blue-purple discoloration of the overlying skin. Angiosarcoma of the breast is an aggressive neoplasm, generally with an extremely poor prognosis. The most important predictor of behavior in this lesion is the degree of tumor differentiation (grade). Well differentiated tumors generally have a somewhat more favorable prognosis, while poorly differentiated ones usually have an unfavorable outcome. This lesion may metastasize to the contralateral breast, as well as to the lungs and various other sites of the body through the bloodstream. Lymph node metastases are extremely rare. The recommended treatment for angiosarcoma is complete surgical resection, which may be combined with chemotherapy and radiotherapy.

IMAGING

The role of mammography in evaluation of *fibroadenoma* is limited. Calcifications in fibroadenoma, when present, most commonly develop in the form of large, coarse calcifications located peripherally and increasing over time. Linear branching calcifications may also occur occasionally and may be similar to those seen in intraductal carcinoma. Ultrasonography may reveal a round or oval mass with a smooth wall and homogeneous internal echoes, but it is not reliable in differentiating benign from malignant solid masses.

Phyllodes tumors appear as well-circumscribed lobular masses with smooth margins on mammography. By ultrasound they are solid with smooth walls, low-level internal echoes, and good through transmission of the sound.

Fibromatosis usually produces a spiculated mass on mammography without calcifications. This appearance may mimic that of carcinoma. The mammographic pattern of *granular cell tumor* is also that of a mass lesion with an ill-defined margin, sometimes with few spiculations which may mimic invasive carcinoma.

Fibrosarcomas present as dense masses with partially indistinct margins. The imaging features of *angiosarcomas* are nonspecific. The lesions usually present as single or multiple masses with indistinct margins. Their sonographic features are also variable; they usually present as solid, multilobulated, poorly circumscribed, inhomogeneous masses. Other types of breast sarcoma have no diagnostic imaging features.

GROSS

Fibroadenomas are well-circumscribed, round to oval, rubbery masses, usually 2–3 cm in size. Some tumors, however, may reach massive proportions (over 10 cm). The cut surfaces are grayish-white, bulging, fleshy, and sometimes glistening and myxoid in appearance. Cleft-like spaces and rare small cysts may be present.

Juvenile fibroadenomas vary in size considerably; some may be very large. They are usually firm on palpation and pinkish-tan in color, with a somewhat nodular appearance on the cut surfaces.

Phyllodes tumors form round or oval masses that are usually sharply circumscribed. Some of them, however, may have bosselated contours. These lesions vary greatly in size, and the size is not a reliable indicator of the biologic behavior. The cut surfaces are usually solid, grayish-white, and fleshy, sometimes even gelatinous in appearance. Clefts, leaf-like processes, and even cystic spaces may be observed on bulging, lobulated, cut surfaces. Areas of necrosis and hemorrhage may be present in the larger lesions.

The gross appearance of the lesions included in the category of *carcinosarcomas* is highly variable. The lesions vary considerably in size and may show circumscribed or irregular margins. On the cut surfaces, fleshy as well as hard areas may be present. Foci of necrosis and hemorrhage may occur in the larger lesions.

Benign mesenchymal proliferations of the breast demonstrate gross appearances similar to those of their counterparts occurring elsewhere in the body. Of special interest in this group are fibromatosis and the granular cell tumors, as both lesions may, at times, resemble infiltrating carcinoma. *Fibromatosis* involving the breast grossly presents as an ill-defined lesion which varies considerably in size (median, 2.5 to 3.0 cm). The lesion, however, is usually soft in consistency and grayish-white to grayish-tan in color on the cut surfaces. The *granular cell tumors* are usually located within the breast tissue proper, but nipple involvement also occurs rarely. These tumors are usually 1 to 2 cm in size. On the cut surfaces some of the lesions appear well circumscribed, but others may have a suspicious irregular margin.

Gross appearances of the *primary sarcomas of the breast* are identical to those of the soft tissue sarcomas occurring in other parts of the body and will not be discussed here in detail. Some of the sarcomas, however, are more often encountered as a component of phyllodes tumor and carcinosarcoma. The *angiosarcomas* of the breast, on the other hand, usually present in a pure form and appear grossly as poorly defined lesions with spongy consistency. The cut surfaces may demonstrate hemorrhagic areas, with a rim of congested vessels surrounding the lesion. The tumor may extend to involve the overlying skin.

35. Fibroadenoma vs Low-Grade Phyllodes Tumor

Fibroadenoma is a benign biphasic tumor of the breast characterized by proliferation of both the stromal and epithelial elements. Two patterns of the lesion are recognized, pericanalicular and intracanalicular. In the pericanalicular pattern there is concentric or random proliferation of the stroma around the ducts (Figs. 35.1 and 35.2), while in the intracanalicular pattern the stromal proliferation, which exhibits a radial growth pattern, is rather prominent and distorts the ducts into elongated and compressed, slit-like spaces (Figs. 35.3 and 35.4). The two patterns may sometimes coexist (Fig. 35.5). In fibroadenomas the epithelial component is composed of two types of cells (epithelial and myoepithelial), as in the normal breast parenchyma. The biphasic (fibroepithelial) nature of fibroadenoma will also be observed in fine needle aspiration preparations (Fig. 35.6). The stroma of fibroadenomas may show variable hypercellularity. Those lesions with hypercellular stroma but with no evidence of a prominent leaf-like growth pattern are referred to as *"cellular fibroadenomas"* (Fig. 35.7). Some lesions, on the other hand, may show dominance of the stroma over the epithelial elements, with formation of a leaf-like pattern but without significant stromal hypercellularity. Tavassoli refers to these lesions with an exaggerated intracanalicular pattern as *"fibroadenoma phyllodes"* (Fig. 35.8). These lesions, however, are probably included in the benign or low-grade phyllodes tumor categories in other classifications. Fibroadenomas are usually well circumscribed but rarely encapsulated. Some lesions may have an irregular periphery.

A variety of secondary alterations may be seen in fibroadenomas, and these may involve the epithelial or stromal components. Fibrocystic changes including cyst formation and adenosis may occur, the latter in up to 10% of the cases (Figs. 35.9 and 35.10). Metaplastic alterations such as squamous and apocrine metaplasia may be observed in 10–15% of the cases (Figs. 35.9 and 35.11). Epithelial hyperplastic changes with or without atypia may also occur in fibroadenomas (Fig. 35.12), as well as hyperplasia and prominent myoid transformation of the myoepithelial cells. CIS of both the lobular and ductal types may arise in fibroadenomas, the former more frequently (Figs. 35.13–35.16). Rarely, the two types of in situ carcinoma may coexist. In approximately 20% of these cases there is an associated CIS in the adjacent stroma. Various types of infiltrating carcinoma have also been observed arising in fi-

broadenomas, as well as secondary involvement of fibroadenoma by an invasive carcinoma from the adjacent breast tissue.

Various alterations may also take place in the stroma of fibroadenomas. Myxoid change, hyalinization, and calcification may be present. Metaplastic stromal changes in the form of osteoid, chondroid, and smooth muscle metaplasia may also occur. Atypical and bizarre, multinucleated giant cells, similar to those sometimes observed in the mammary stroma with fibrocystic changes, are occasionally identified in the stroma of fibroadenomas. These cells have no prognostic significance and should not be mistaken for malignant cells. Sarcomas may develop in fibroadenomas, but very rarely. Another secondary alteration that may be observed in fibroadenomas is spontaneous infarction, which usually occurs during pregnancy and lactation.

Phyllodes tumor, the second well-recognized biphasic tumor of the breast, is composed of benign epithelial elements and cellular spindle cell stroma. The characteristic feature of this lesion is the formation of leaf-like processes often protruding into cyst-like spaces (Figs. 35.17 and 35.18). The epithelial component of phyllodes tumor is composed of the usual two cell types characteristic of the mammary ductal-lobular system, as in fibroadenoma. The stroma of the phyllodes tumors, on the other hand, is more densely cellular than that of fibroadenoma and often has a fibrosarcomatous appearance (Figs. 35.17–35.20). Diagnostic features of phyllodes tumor may also be observed in core needle biopsies (Fig. 35.21) and fine needle aspiration preparations (Fig. 35.22). Phyllodes tumors may have pushing or infiltrating borders. Even in those tumors that grossly appear circumscribed, the margin may infiltrate adjacent breast tissue.

Secondary alterations similar to those seen in fibroadenoma may also occur in phyllodes tumor. These include fibrocystic changes such as metaplastic alterations, adenosis (Figs. 35.23 and 35.24), and epithelial hyperplasia with or without atypia. In situ and infiltrating carcinomas of both the lobular and ductal type may also occur in phyllodes tumor (Figs. 35.25 and 35.26), but much less commonly than in fibroadenomas. Although the stroma of phyllodes tumor is composed mainly of spindle-shaped fibroblasts, lipoid, chondroid, osteoid, smooth muscle, and rhabdomyoblastic differentiation may occur. If the stroma is clearly malignant, it is often fibrosarcomatous (Figs. 35.27 and 35.28).

However, various other types of soft tissue sarcomas may also develop in phyllodes tumor, including liposarcoma (Figs. 35.29 and 35.30), chondrosarcoma, osteogenic sarcoma, and rhabdomyosarcoma. Mixed types of differentiation also occur, making classification of the sarcomatous component difficult. Sarcomatous stromal overgrowth, which is a poor prognostic sign, may also occur in some cases of phyllodes tumor.

The differentiation of ordinary *intracanalicular fibroadenoma* from *low-grade phyllodes tumor* is usually not difficult. The low-grade phyllodes tumors characteristically form leaf-like processes protruding into cystic spaces (exaggerated intracanalicular growth pattern) and, as a rule, their stroma is more cellular than that of fibroadenoma (Figs. 35.31 and 35.32). In differentiating the *cellular variants of fibroadenoma* from *low-grade phyllodes tumor*, the presence or absence of the well-formed leaf-like growth pattern and the degree of stromal cellularity are the crucial features. If the lesion lacks or shows rare, poorly defined leaf-like processes and the stroma shows only mild or localized hypercellularity, the lesion is designated as cellular fibroadenoma (Fig. 35.33). If the stroma is more cellular than that of fibroadenoma and leaf-like processes are present, the lesion is classified as low-grade phyllodes tumor (Figs. 35.34 and 35.35). If, however, the stromal cellularity is borderline, the presence of a well-formed leaf-like growth pattern, according to Tavassoli, also favors a low-grade phyllodes tumor. If, on the other hand, a well-formed leaf-like pattern is present but the stroma is hypocellular or comparable to that of fibroadenoma, the lesion is referred to as *"fibroadenoma phyllodes"* by Tavassoli and probably placed into benign or low-grade phyllodes tumor categories by others (Fig. 35.36). Some lesions, however, fall into the truly borderline category and may not be easily classifiable. In these cases, especially if the patient is young, the conservative diagnosis of fibroadenoma is recommended.

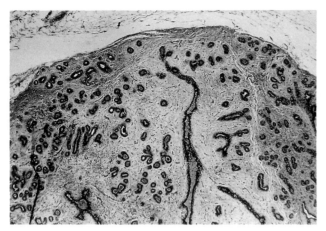

Figure 35.1. Fibroadenoma, pericanalicular pattern.

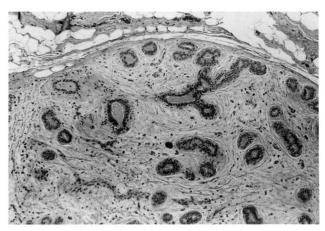

Figure 35.2. Fibroadenoma, pericanalicular pattern.

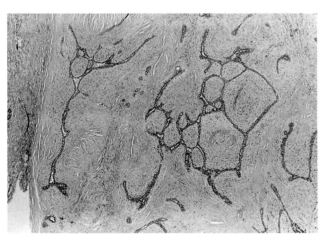

Figure 35.3. Fibroadenoma, intracanalicular pattern.

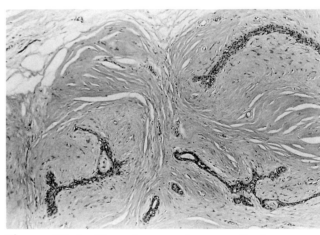

Figure 35.4. Fibroadenoma, intracanalicular pattern.

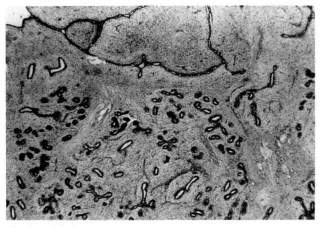

Figure 35.5. Fibroadenoma, mixed pattern.

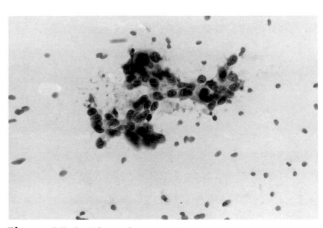

Figure 35.6. Fibroadenoma. FNA.

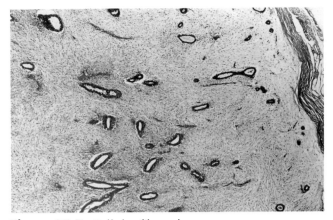

Figure 35.7. Cellular fibroadenoma.

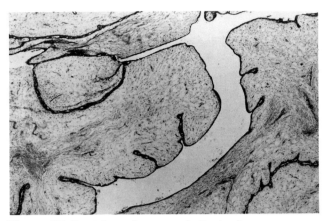

Figure 35.8. "Fibroadenoma phyllodes."

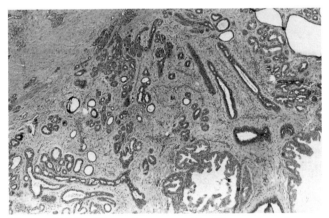

Figure 35.9. Fibroadenoma with fibrocystic changes.

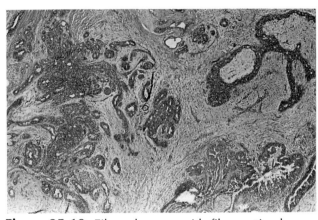

Figure 35.10. Fibroadenoma with fibrocystic changes.

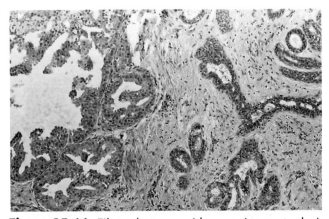

Figure 35.11. Fibroadenoma with apocrine metaplasia.

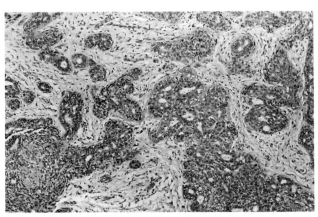

Figure 35.12. Fibroadenoma with usual epithelial hyperplasia.

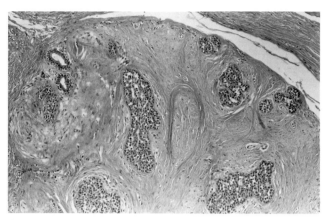

Figure 35.13. Lobular carcinoma in situ in fibroadenoma.

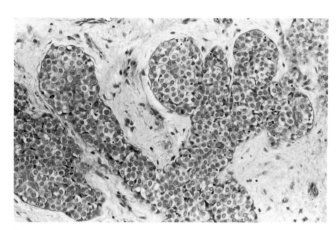

Figure 35.14. Lobular carcinoma in situ in fibroadenoma.

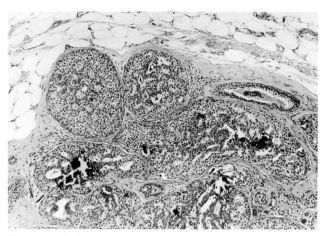

Figure 35.15. Ductal carcinoma in situ in fibroadenoma.

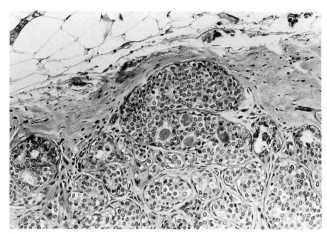

Figure 35.16. Ductal carcinoma in situ in fibroadenoma.

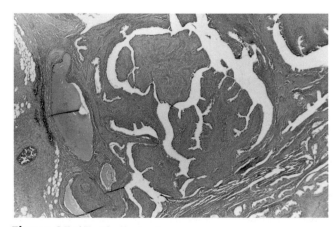

Figure 35.17. Phyllodes tumor.

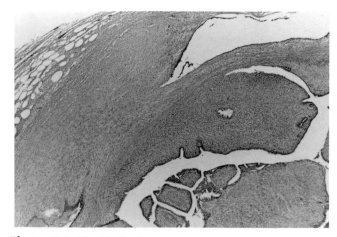

Figure 35.18. Phyllodes tumor.

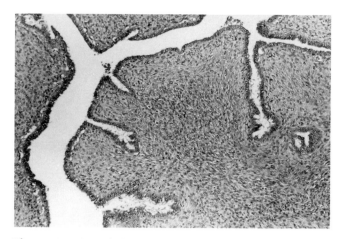

Figure 35.19. Phyllodes tumor.

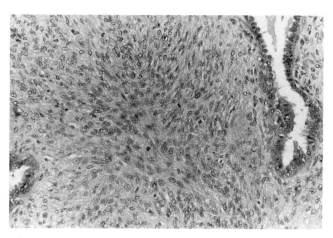

Figure 35.20. Phyllodes tumor.

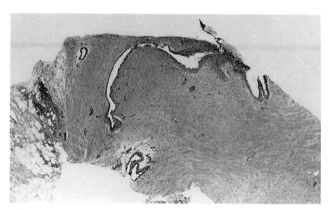

Figure 35.21. Phyllodes tumor, core needle biopsy.

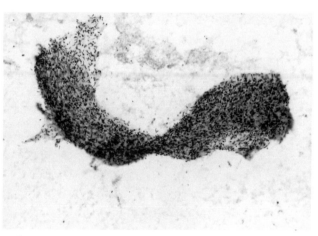

Figure 35.22. Phyllodes tumor. FNA.

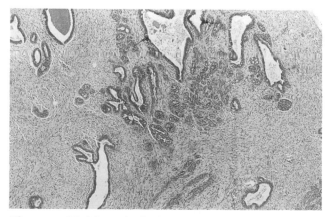

Figure 35.23. Phyllodes tumor with fibrocystic changes.

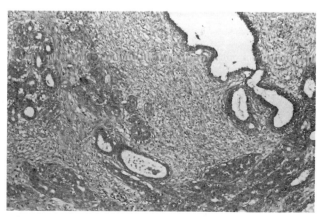

Figure 35.24. Phyllodes tumor with fibrocystic changes.

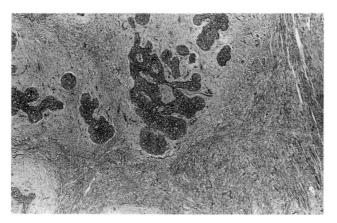

Figure 35.25. Lobular carcinoma in situ in phyllodes tumor.

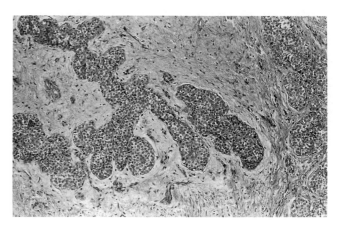

Figure 35.26. Lobular carcinoma in situ in phyllodes tumor.

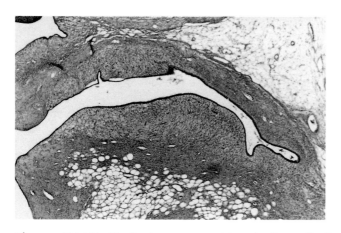

Figure 35.27. Phyllodes tumor with spindle cell (fibrosarcomatous) stroma.

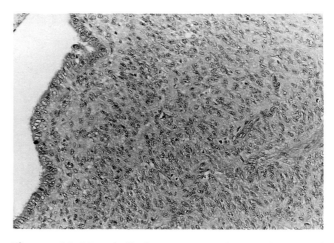

Figure 35.28. Phyllodes tumor with spindle cell (fibrosarcomatous) stroma.

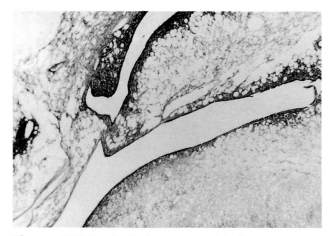

Figure 35.29. Phyllodes tumor with liposarcomatous stroma.

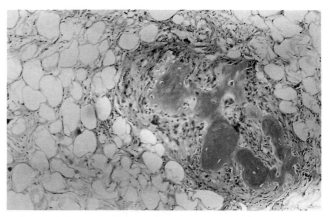

Figure 35.30. Liposarcomatous stroma with osseous metaplasia, phyllodes tumor.

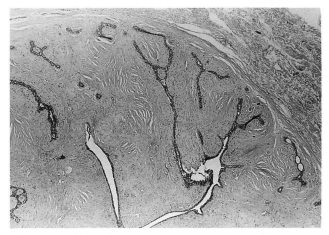

Figure 35.31. Fibroadenoma, intracanalicular type.

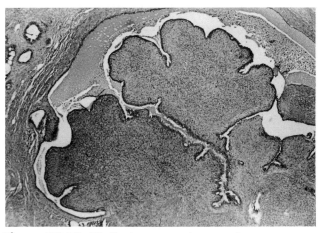

Figure 35.32. Phyllodes tumor, low grade.

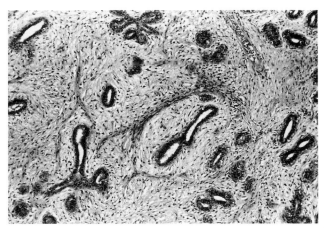

Figure 35.33. Cellular fibroadenoma.

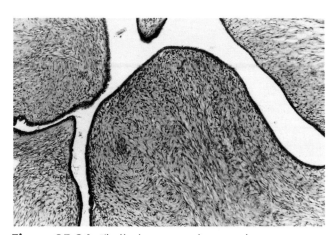

Figure 35.34. Phyllodes tumor, low grade.

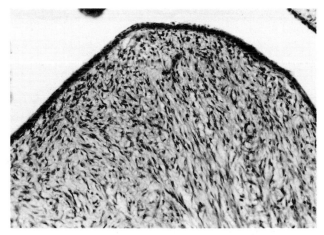

Figure 35.35. Phyllodes tumor, low grade.

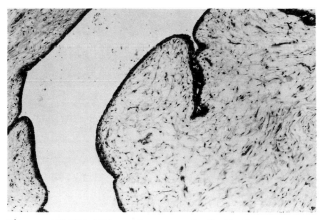

Figure 35.36. "Fibroadenoma phyllodes."

36. Juvenile Fibroadenoma vs Fibroadenoma of the Adult Type vs Low-Grade Phyllodes Tumor

Juvenile fibroadenoma is a distinctive biphasic tumor of the breast. The lesion usually, but not always, displays a pericanalicular growth pattern. These lesions are composed of irregularly proliferating ductal structures, often with epithelial hyperplastic changes, surrounded by a stroma which is dense and cellular (Fig. 36.1)

In differentiating *juvenile fibroadenoma* from *fibroadenoma of the adult type*, the cellularity of the stroma, which is usually more prominent in juvenile fibroadenoma than that of the adult type, is the most important feature (Figs. 36.1–36.4). The rarity of the intracanalicular growth pattern in juvenile fibroadenoma is an additional helpful feature in this differentiation (Figs. 36.1 and 36.3).

In distinguishing the *juvenile fibroadenoma* from the *low-grade phyllodes tumor*, recognition of the typical leaf-like growth pattern of phyllodes tumor is most important (Figs. 36.5 and 36.6). In addition, the stroma is usually much more cellular in phyllodes tumor than in juvenile fibroadenoma (Figs. 36.5 and 36.6), and the patients with phyllodes tumor are usually older. This distinction is very important, since in adolescent patients with juvenile fibroadenoma the excision should spare as much of the adjacent breast tissue as possible, while in those with phyllodes tumor, total removal with wider excision is recommended to prevent local recurrences.

Presentation as a discrete mass lesion differentiates *juvenile fibroadenoma* from *juvenile hypertrophy*, which usually causes diffuse enlargement of the entire breast.

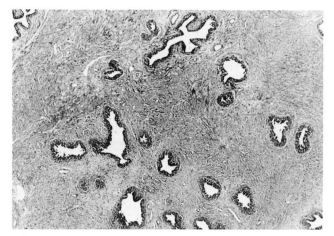

Figure 36.1. Juvenile fibroadenoma.

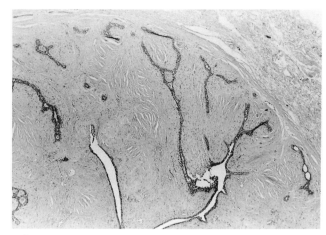

Figure 36.2. Fibroadenoma.

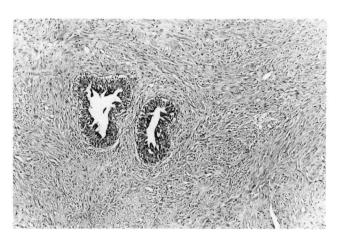

Figure 36.3. Juvenile fibroadenoma.

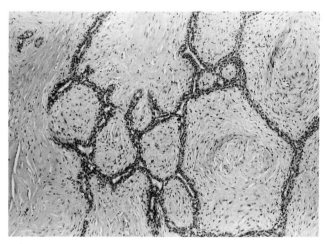

Figure 36.4. Fibroadenoma.

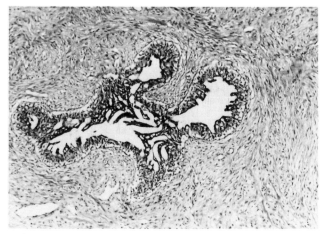

Figure 36.5. Juvenile fibroadenoma.

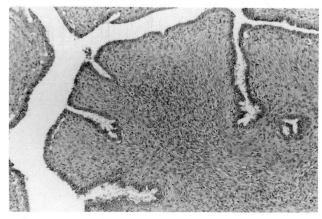

Figure 36.6. Phyllodes tumor.

37. Fibroadenoma with Superimposed Sclerosing Adenosis vs Fibroadenoma with Infiltrating Carcinoma

Another problem which may be encountered with fibroadenoma is the differentiation of *sclerosing adenosis occurring in fibroadenoma* (Fig. 37.1) from *infiltrating ductal carcinoma involving fibroadenoma*, specifically the tubular type (Fig. 37.2). The presence of the myoepithelial cells and basement membrane around the proliferating and distorted ductules of sclerosing adenosis occurring in fibroadenoma identifies their benign nature (Fig. 37.1). If necessary, a PAS stain and immunoperoxidase stains for actin may be performed to help demonstrate the presence of the basement membrane and the myoepithelial cells in the distorted ductules in question. Careful evaluation of the overall histologic features is also essential in making this distinction.

On rare occasions, markedly compressed ductular units of *sclerosing adenosis with very little or no resid-ual lumen occurring in fibroadenoma* may mimic *infiltrating lobular carcinoma involving fibroadenoma* (Figs. 37.3–37.6). In this form of adenosis, which largely lacks evident ductules, the persistent epithelial elements are usually the spindled myoepithelial cells with uniform nuclei (Figs. 37.3 and 37.5). The classical infiltrating lobular carcinoma, on the other hand, is composed of rounded cells arranged in rigid linear arrays (Figs. 37.4 and 37.6). The absence of CIS within fibroadenoma and/or in the adjacent breast parenchyma also supports the benign nature of the process. If necessary, immunohistochemistry may also be used in making this distinction. Differentiation of sclerosing adenosis, with or without marked ductular attenuation from tubular and infiltrating lobular carcinoma, respectively, was also discussed in more detail in Section 1.

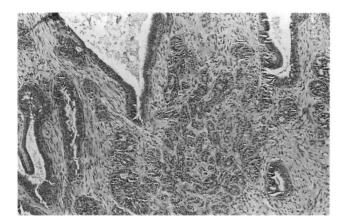

Figure 37.1. Adenosis in fibroadenoma.

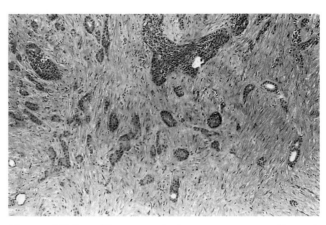

Figure 37.2. Infiltrating tubular carcinoma in fibroadenoma.

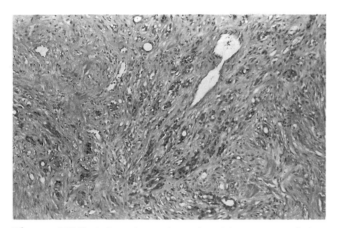

Figure 37.3. Sclerosing adenosis with attenuated ductules in fibroadenoma.

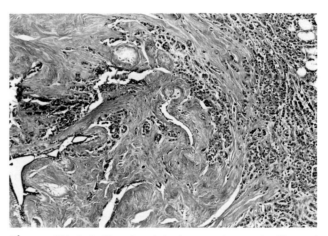

Figure 37.4. Infiltrating lobular carcinoma in fibroadenoma.

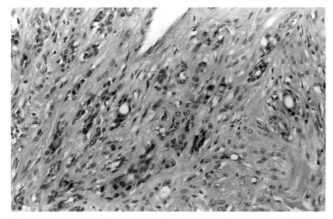

Figure 37.5. Sclerosing adenosis with attenuated ductules in fibroadenoma.

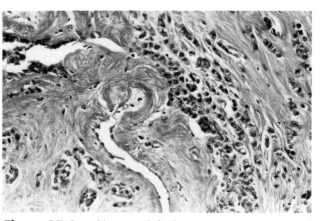

Figure 37.6. Infiltrating lobular carcinoma in fibroadenoma.

38. Low-Grade (Benign) Phyllodes Tumor vs High-Grade (Malignant) Phyllodes Tumor

The classification of the *phyllodes tumors* (a generic term proposed by the World Health Organization) and opinions concerning the prognostic significance of the morphologic features of this group of lesions have been variable. The current terminology is also not uniform, since the term *cystosarcoma phyllodes (CP)*, continues to be widely used for this group of lesions. Many pathologists who use this term divide the lesions into benign and malignant categories, based mainly upon the microscopic features of the stroma. They consider the lesion *malignant* if the stroma has features resembling those of the soft tissue sarcomas and histologically *benign* if the stroma has no malignant features. Norris and Taylor, who also used the designation *cystosarcoma phyllodes*, concluded in their review article that no single histologic feature could reliably predict the behavior of these tumors and that each lesion should be evaluated individually based on the combination of tumor size, tumor margin, cytologic atypia, and mitotic activity. Other investigators, referring to the lesions as either *cystosarcoma phyllodes* or *phyllodes tumor*, have proposed separating them into *benign*, *intermediate* (borderline), and *malignant* categories based on the composite evaluation of various features. Their criteria, however, have been variable, and the intermediate (borderline) group appears to have no definite predictive value. Based on this conclusion, recognition of *benign* and *malignant forms* of CP with subdivision of the malignant group into the *low-grade* and *high-grade* categories has been proposed, placing most of the borderline lesions into the low-grade category.

At AFIP, where the term *cystosarcoma phyllodes* is also preferred, the lesions are divided into *low-grade* and *high-grade* categories, with the low-grade lesions having a tendency toward local recurrence and the high grade lesions having potential for metastases. The qualifications of benign and malignant are not used for CP at AFIP, since the accurate prediction of recurrences and/or metastases is usually not possible, and even the histologically benign lesions are capable of at least recurrence. It appears, however, that Tavassoli excludes the lesions with a well-formed leaf-like growth pattern, but with hypocellular stroma or stroma comparable to that of fibroadenoma, from the category of CP and refers to these lesions as *"fibroadenoma phyllodes."* These lesions are probably included in the benign or low-grade phyllodes tumor categories in other classifications (Figs. 35.8 and 35.36). For the distinction between the *low-grade* and *high-grade* tumors, Tavassoli recommends utilization of the criteria proposed earlier by Norris and Taylor. Tumors with predominantly pushing margins, mild to moderate atypia, and fewer than three mitotic figures per 10 high-power fields (HPF) are considered low grade, with potential for local recurrence but very little tendency to metastasize (Figs. 38.1 and 38.2). Those tumors with infiltrating or pushing margins, moderate to severe atypia, and three or more mitotic figures per 10 HPF are considered high grade, with potential for distant metastases (Figs. 38.3–38.6). If a specific type of sarcoma component is present within the stroma of the phyllodes tumor, this should also be included in the diagnosis (see Figs. 35.29 and 35.30). Sarcomatous overgrowth is an additional factor which is considered a significant morphologic indicator of malignant behavior in phyllodes tumors. Therefore, the phyllodes tumors showing sarcomatous overgrowth, with only a minor residual phyllodes tumor component recognizable, are also placed in the high-grade category (see Chapter 39).

Flow cytometry has been evaluated as a predictive tool in phyllodes tumor. Although DNA content (ploidy) and proliferative rate (S-phase) have been found to correlate with outcome independent of histology by some authors, others have demonstrated conflicting results, mainly with DNA ploidy.

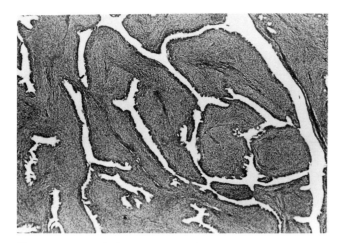

Figure 38.1. Phyllodes tumor, low grade.

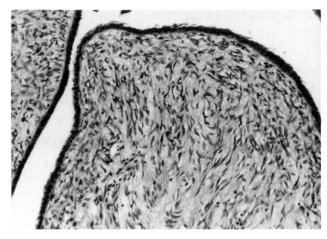

Figure 38.2. Phyllodes tumor, low grade.

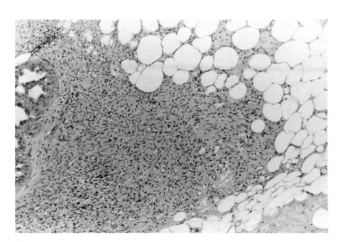

Figure 38.3. Phyllodes tumor, high grade.

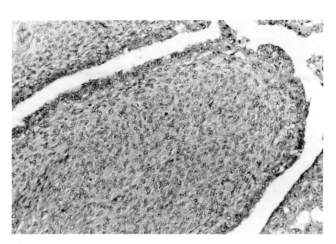

Figure 38.4. Phyllodes tumor, high grade.

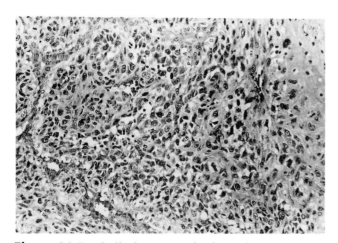

Figure 38.5. Phyllodes tumor, high grade.

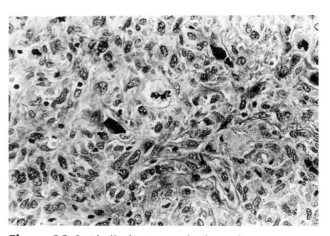

Figure 38.6. Phyllodes tumor, high grade.

39. High-Grade Phyllodes Tumor with Sarcomatous Overgrowth vs Pure Sarcoma

Although the aggressive stromal component of the *high-grade phyllodes tumors* is usually a spindle cell sarcoma with fibrosarcomatous features, other specific types of sarcoma such as liposarcoma, chondrosarcoma, osteogenic sarcoma, rhabdomyosarcoma, and malignant fibrous histiocytoma can also develop in these tumors (Figs. 35.29 and 35.30, 39.1–39.6) (see also Chapters 35 and 38).

Primary breast sarcomas are morphologically identical to the soft tissue sarcomas occurring in other parts of the body. Although most of these lesions, except angiosarcoma, more often occur as a component of phyllodes tumor or carcinosarcoma, they may also be seen in a pure form. After diagnosis and proper classification, the sarcomas of the breast are graded (based on the mitotic count, pleomorphism, cellularity, type of margins, and the presence or absence of necrosis) into low-, intermediate-, and high-grade categories like their soft tissue counterparts.

If there is extensive *overgrowth* by any type of *sarcoma within a phyllodes tumor*, distinction of the lesion from *pure breast sarcoma* may be difficult. In these cases, careful examination and adequate sampling of the tumor is necessary, since the epithelial component in some of these large tumors with sarcomatous overgrowth may be reduced significantly, becoming barely identifiable (Fig. 39.1).

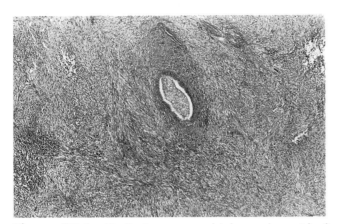

Figure 39.1. Phyllodes tumor, high grade, with fibrosarcomatous overgrowth.

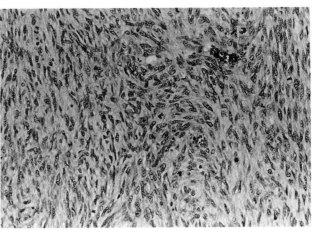

Figure 39.2. Phyllodes tumor, high grade, with fibrosarcomatous overgrowth.

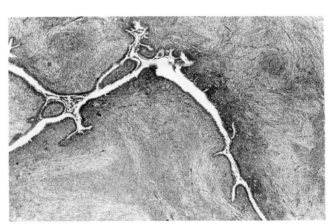

Figure 39.3. Phyllodes tumor, high grade, with fibrosarcomatous overgrowth.

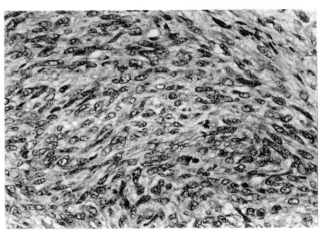

Figure 39.4. Phyllodes tumor, high grade, with fibrosarcomatous overgrowth.

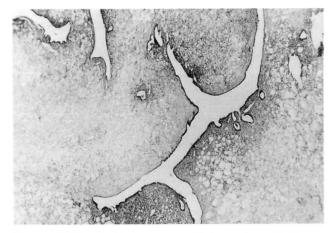

Figure 39.5. Phyllodes tumor, high grade, with liposarcomatous overgrowth.

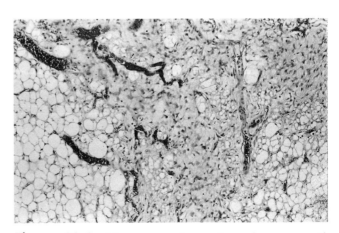

Figure 39.6. Liposarcomatous stromal overgrowth, phyllodes tumor, high grade.

40. Periductal Stromal Sarcoma vs Phyllodes Tumor vs Pure Sarcoma

Hypercellular periductal stromal tumor, cellular periductal stromal tumor, periductal stromal tumor, and periductal sarcoma are the terms earlier utilized or proposed by various authors as alternate designations for the phyllodes tumor. Tavassoli, on the other hand, uses the term *"periductal stromal sarcoma"* for a specific biphasic breast tumor characterized by tubules with open lumina surrounded by cellular sarcomatous spindle cell proliferation forming periductal nodules. The nodules are often separated by adipose tissue aggregates. In differentiating the *periductal stromal sarcoma*, a lesion which is not widely recognized as a distinct entity, from the *phyllodes tumor*, the absence of a leaf-like growth pattern, which is characteristic of phyllodes tumor (Figs. 40.1–40.4), is the most important feature.

The distinct periductal nature of the proliferation with a typical nodular growth pattern differentiates *periductal stromal sarcoma* from the *pure spindle cell sarcomas* of the breast (Figs. 40.5 and 40.6).

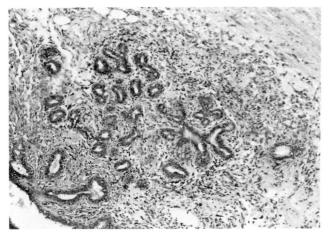

Figure 40.1. Periductal stromal sarcoma.

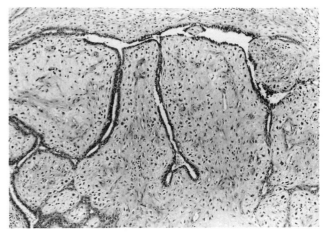

Figure 40.2. Phyllodes tumor.

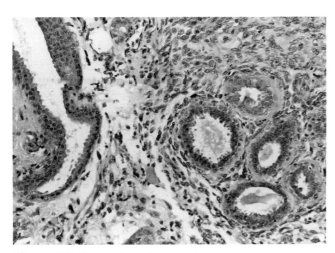

Figure 40.3. Periductal stromal sarcoma.

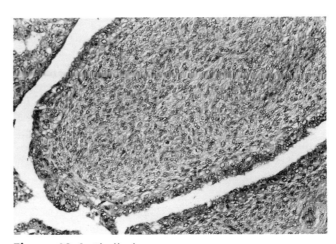

Figure 40.4. Phyllodes tumor.

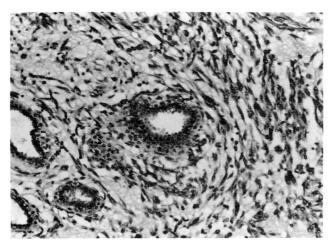

Figure 40.5. Periductal stromal sarcoma.

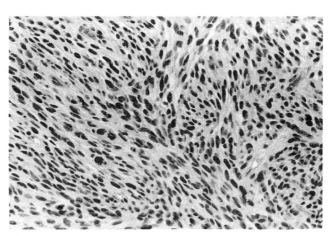

Figure 40.6. Pure spindle cell sarcoma.

41. Carcinosarcoma vs Metaplastic Carcinoma vs Pure Sarcoma

Carcinosarcoma is a rare biphasic tumor which consists of malignant epithelial and mesenchymal components. True carcinosarcomas of the breast are exceedingly uncommon and are not well defined. According to Tavassoli, two main groups of lesions qualify for this designation: high-grade phyllodes tumors containing a carcinomatous component and biphasic malignant tumors that have no phyllodes tumor in the background. A rare primary synovial sarcoma of the breast is also included in the category of carcinosarcomas of the breast by Tavassoli. The lesions in the first group may also be designated as carcinomas arising in phyllodes tumors. The second group of lesions are considered by Tavassoli to be metaplastic, and of epithelial or myoepithelial origin. Many experts, on the other hand, consider the lesions in this category carcinomas with metaplasia (metaplastic carcinomas) and refer only to those lesions with a background of phyllodes tumor as carcinosarcomas. Rare collision tumors are also included in the category of carcinosarcoma by some authors. Although poorly differentiated infiltrating ductal carcinoma is the most common, any type of carcinoma may constitute a carcinomatous component of lesions classified as carcinosarcoma by Tavassoli and as metaplastic carcinoma by others. The sarcomatous component of the lesion may be in the form of any of the soft tissue sarcomas. In the lesions classified as *carcinosarcoma* by Tavassoli, a positive immunostaining reaction for cytokeratin is observed in the carcinomatous component, whereas the sarcomatous component demonstrates positive immunostaining for a variety of mesenchymal antigens but not for cytokeratin. *Metaplastic carcinomas*, according to most other authorities, represent a heterogeneous group of neoplasms which demonstrate an admixture of adenocarcinoma with squamous, spindle cell (pseudosarcomatous), and heterologous (chondroid, osteoid, etc.) metaplastic components (Figs. 41.1–41.6). The amount and differentiation of various metaplastic components within the tumors are highly variable. Tavassoli, on the other hand, recognizes their metaplastic nature but includes most of these lesions in the carcinosarcoma category, and considers only those lesions with demonstrable epithelial antigens in the sarcomatous-appearing areas to be *metaplastic carcinomas*.

Therefore, if Tavassoli's classification is followed, routine light microscopy as well as immunohistochemistry should be used to distinguish between *carcinosarcoma* and *metaplastic carcinoma*. Ultrastructural study may be of additional help. In all tumors with a clear-cut or suggestive malignant biphasic pattern, Tavassoli recommends the use of immunoperoxidase stains for cytokeratin and various mesenchymal antigens (actin, vimentin, etc.). If positive immunoperoxidase staining for cytokeratin is observed in the sarcomatous-appearing areas of the tumor, she considers the lesion metaplastic carcinoma (Figs. 41.3–41.6). If, on the other hand, no positive staining is present for cytokeratin in any of the sarcomatous components, then she classifies the lesion as carcinosarcoma. If the classification of other experts is followed, the distinction of lesions designated as carcinosarcoma (in which carcinomatous and sarcomatous elements can be traced separately to epithelial and mesenchymal origins such as carcinomas arising in high-grade phyllodes tumors) from metaplastic carcinoma is usually not difficult.

Some of the *carcinomas with squamous metaplasia* may assume a predominantly *spindle cell* (pseudosarcomatous) growth pattern. These tumors may mimic *pure spindle cell sarcomas* of the breast (Figs. 41.3–41.6). Extensive sampling is necessary in these tumors to locate the squamous differentiation and foci of in situ or invasive carcinoma (Figs. 41.3 and 41.5). Immunohistochemistry (Fig. 41.6) and electron microscopy offer further help in making this distinction. The differential diagnostic problems associated with this heterologous group of lesions are discussed further in Section 5.

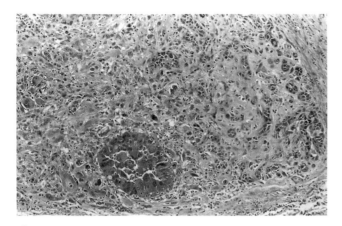

Figure 41.1. Metaplastic carcinoma.

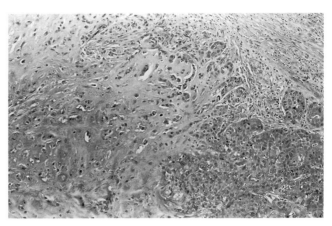

Figure 41.2. Metaplastic carcinoma.

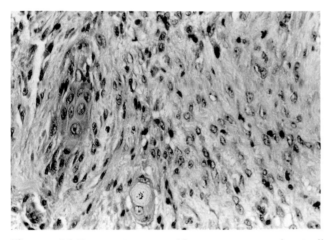

Figure 41.3. Carcinoma with squamous and spindle cell metaplasia.

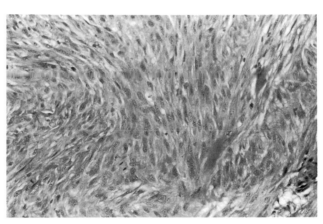

Figure 41.4. Carcinoma with prominent spindle cell metaplasia.

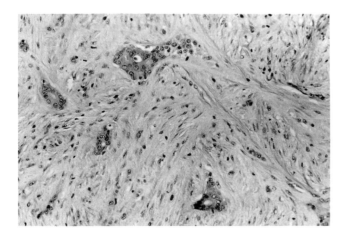

Figure 41.5. Carcinoma with spindle cell metaplasia.

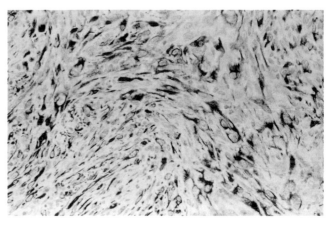

Figure 41.6. Carcinoma with prominent spindle cell metaplasia, cytokeratin immunoperoxidase.

42. Pseudoangiomatous Hyperplasia of Mammary Stroma vs Angiosarcoma

Pseudoangiomatous hyperplasia of the mammary stroma (PHMS) is characterized by a dense collagenous proliferation of the mammary stroma containing an interanastomosing pattern of slit-like spaces (Figs. 42.1–42.3). The lesion is frequently seen as an incidental microscopic finding in breast biopsies performed for a variety of benign or malignant lesions. It also occurs as a discrete mass lesion, however, as was described in its original reporting. In PHMS the stromal cells bordering the anastomosing slit-like spaces are flat, discontinuous, and inconspicuous. The intervening dense collagen often appears hyalinized and keloid-like. These changes, although more prominent in intralobular stroma and often seen immediately surrounding lobules in a concentric fashion, also extend into the interlobular stroma. Powell et al. recently described the proliferative variants of this lesion with increased stromal cellularity which largely obscured the pseudoangiomatous lumina. Even in these cases, however, areas with a typical pseudoangiomatous pattern could be easily identified. The ultrastructural and immunohistochemical studies were also performed by Powell et al. on both the usual and proliferative variants of the lesion, demonstrating findings consistent with myofibroblastic histogenesis.

Angiosarcomas of the breast are composed of open, anastomosing vascular channels lined by endothelial cells, either single or multilayered, also forming tufts, papillae, and solid spindle cell areas in various proportions, depending on the differentiation of the lesion (Figs. 42.4–42.6). The endothelial cells are usually plump and hyperchromatic, showing varying degrees of atypia and mitotic activity. Studies done by different groups demonstrated that the grading of angiosarcomas based on the differentiation correlates with the prognosis. As a result, various grading protocols have been proposed, dividing the lesions into well, moderately, and poorly differentiated types; low, intermediate, and high grades; and type I, type II and type III categories, all based on the differentiation. Of these classifications, that of Merino and associates, which utilizes a quantitative approach to the grading and divides the lesions into well, moderately, and poorly differentiated categories, appears to be the most applicable. According to this classification, one to two layers of endothelial cells lining well-formed anastomosing vascular channels and showing rare mitotic figures are the diagnostic features of the well-differentiated category. In the moderately differentiated category, solid spindle cell areas are present, comprising less than 20% of the total tumor mass. In contrast, the poorly differentiated lesions are composed predominantly of solid spindle cell nests, with marked cellular pleomorphism, mitoses, and areas of necrosis.

It is not difficult to distinguish poorly and moderately differentiated angiosarcomas from PHMS, but problems may rarely be encountered with the well-differentiated lesions. In *PHMS* the anastomosing spaces are narrow and slit-like (Figs. 42.1–42.3), rather than well formed and open, as in *well-differentiated angiosarcoma* (Figs. 42.4–42.6), and they are lobulocentric in distribution. *PHMS* merges with intralobular stroma and extends into the interlobular stroma, but the lesion does not infiltrate and destroy the lobules and does not invade the fat, as is usually seen in *angiosarcoma*. In *PHMS* the nuclei of the spindle cells lining the slit-like spaces are attenuated, lack atypia, and do not show mitotic activity (Figs. 42.2 and 42.3). In well-differentiated *angiosarcoma*, on the other hand, well-formed interanastomosing vascular channels are lined by one or two layers of endothelial cells which show minimal tufting and rare mitotic figures (Figs. 42.5 and 42.6). In addition, in *PHMS* immunohistochemical studies demonstrate the myofibroblastic nature of the spindle cells. In *angiosarcoma* the endothelial nature of the cells can be demonstrated by a positive reaction for factor VIII–related antigen (F VIII-RA), CD31, and CD34 immunoperoxidase stains, particularly in most of the well-differentiated lesions. The ultrastructural studies are also helpful in making this distinction.

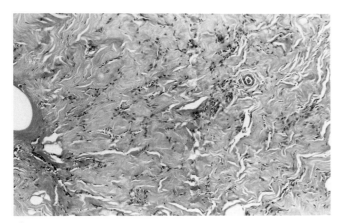

Figure 42.1. Pseudoangiomatous hyperplasia of mammary stroma.

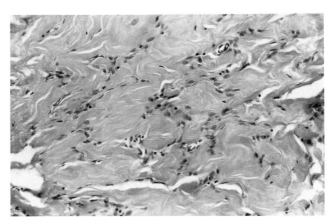

Figure 42.2. Pseudoangiomatous hyperplasia of mammary stroma.

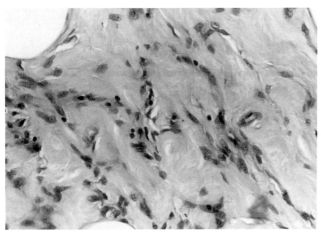

Figure 42.3. Pseudoangiomatous hyperplasia of mammary stroma.

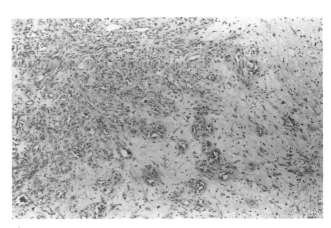

Figure 42.4. Angiosarcoma.

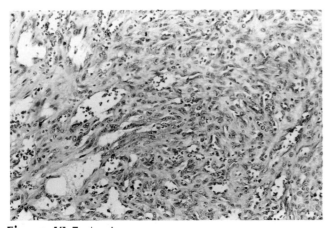

Figure 42.5. Angiosarcoma.

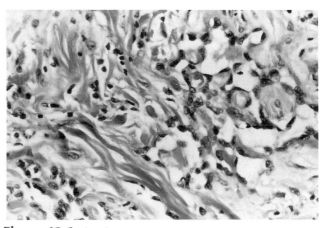

Figure 42.6. Angiosarcoma.

43. Benign Vascular Proliferations vs Angiosarcoma

Vascular tumors of the breast are rare, and the majority are malignant. However, a variety of benign vascular lesions also occur in the breast. These include microscopic perilobular hemangiomas and various other types of hemangiomas (juvenile, capillary, cavernous, and venous types), as well as angiolipoma, angiomatosis, hemangiopericytoma, and papillary endothelial hyperplasia. Some of these benign vascular lesions, however, can mimic angiosarcoma and may pose significant problems in differential diagnosis, mainly because they occur predominantly in the soft tissues and are rather rare in the breast.

The so-called *perilobular hemangiomas* are rather common incidental findings in the breast. They are microscopic lesions that range in size from 0.5 to 4.0 mm. They may be solitary or multiple; bilateral cases also occur. These lesions, however, are not always perilobular in location. They may also be periductal and may extend into the intralobular or interlobular stroma. The perilobular hemangiomas are composed of small vascular channels which vary slightly in size, and they are usually lined by endothelial cells showing no evidence of atypia or pleomorphism. *Other forms of hemangioma* (cavernous, capillary, juvenile, and venous) and benign vascular proliferations are usually larger than 0.5 cm in diameter and are histologically identical to their soft tissue counterparts.

Angiolipomas may involve the breast parenchyma or the subcutaneous tissue. They are composed of mature adipose tissue and collections of small vascular structures. Although their capsule is often not apparent in histologic sections, they are usually rather sharply circumscribed.

Angiomatosis is a very rare vascular lesion in the breast. It is characterized by irregular proliferation of vascular channels lines by endothelial cells showing no evidence of atypia. Vascular channels grow diffusely and surround the ducts and lobules, but extension into and disruption of the lobules are usually not seen. The margins of the lesion are irregular, but the vascular channels are distributed rather uniformly throughout the lesion, without much variation in the pattern.

Papillary endothelial hyperplasia usually occurs intravascularly within the lumina of the preexisting vessels, in hemangiomas and pyogenic granulomas. Occasionally the lesions may occur extravascularly as a result of organizing hematoma. These lesions demonstrate papillary fibroepithelial processes and anastomosing vascular channels. In the region of the breast, they may occur in the breast parenchyma or in the subcutaneous tissue of the breast.

Various types of *hemangiomas* involving the breast should be distinguished from *well-differentiated angiosarcoma*. In general, hemangiomas of the breast are sharply demarcated from the surrounding breast tissue (Fig. 43.1), unlike the angiosarcomas, which have ill-defined margins and infiltrate the surrounding breast parenchyma and adipose tissue in a diffuse, irregular fashion (Fig. 43.2). In addition, the vessels within hemangiomas are often more uniform in size, and there is usually no significant endothelial hyperplasia or atypia. When any of these various types of hemangiomas have cytologic atypia, somewhat irregular margins, and rare foci of anastomosing channels, the term *atypical hemangioma* is applied. These lesions, however, are also small, demonstrate the overall characteristics of various types of benign hemangiomas, and lack the endothelial proliferation, mitotic activity, and extensive vascular anastomoses that characterize the *angiosarcomas*.

Angiolipoma, which is composed of mature adipose tissue and collections of small vessels, should also be distinguished from *angiosarcoma*. Like lipomas, these lesions are sharply circumscribed, and some of the vascular spaces within them may contain microthrombi. Angiolipomas displace the breast parenchyma but do not infiltrate the lobules, as do angiosarcomas. In addition, the vascular component of angiolipomas lacks endothelial hyperplasia and atypia (Figs. 43.3 and 43.4). On careful evaluation of the overall histologic pattern, these lesions are not difficult to differentiate from angiosarcoma (Figs. 43.5 and 43.6).

Angiomatosis may sometimes be difficult to distinguish from *angiosarcoma*, mainly because of its large size and some of its histologic features. These lesions may diffusely infiltrate the breast parenchyma and may show anastomosing vascular channels focally, but their thin-walled, empty vascular channels have flat, bland endothelial cells and lack many of the diagnostic features of moderately and poorly differentiated angiosarcomas such as necrosis, mitotic activity, tufting, and formation of solid sheets. The distinction of *angiomatosis* from *well-differentiated angiosarcoma*, however, may be difficult, especially if only a biopsy is available. In questionable cases, numerous sections should be examined. Angiomatosis usually shows a uniform distribution of vascular spaces, does not show disruption of the lobules, and, for the most part, lacks anastomosing channels and endothelial atypia, while well-differentiated angiosarcoma shows a heterogeneous distribution, infiltrates and disrupts the lobules, and demonstrates prominent anastomosing channels and variable but generally mild endothelial atypia.

Papillary endothelial hyperplasia may also be mistaken for a *well-differentiated angiosarcoma* because of the exuberant nature of the endothelial proliferation, which forms a complex papillary growth pattern and anastomosing vascular channels (Figs. 43.7 and 43.8). This distinction is most difficult, especially if one is dealing with an incisional or needle biopsy. In these instances, and when there is any doubt, complete excision and histologic examination of the lesion should be performed before a final diagnosis is rendered. Intravas-

cular papillary endothelial hyperplasia usually shows a fibrous pseudocapsule, and elastic and muscular tissue of the vascular wall may be demonstrated, by special stains if necessary, proving its intravascular location (Figs. 43.7 and 43.8). The presence of residual thrombotic material intimately associated with vascular proliferation is an additional clue (Fig. 43.8). If the lesion forms within a hemangioma or extravascularly in the soft tissue, the presence of the residual features of the hemangioma or of a preexisting blood clot within the lesion, respectively, will help to identify the benign nature of the process. When these features of the lesion are observed on careful histologic examination (including low-power examination), it is not difficult to distinguish it from well-differentiated angiosarcoma (Figs. 43.5 and 43.6).

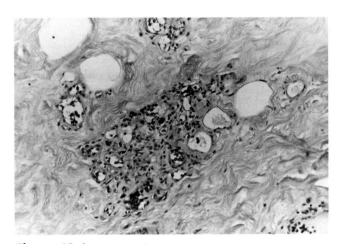

Figure 43.1. Hemangioma.

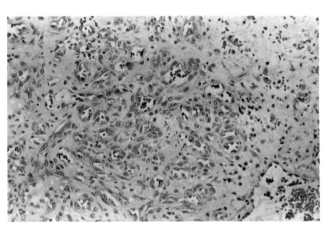

Figure 43.2. Angiosarcoma.

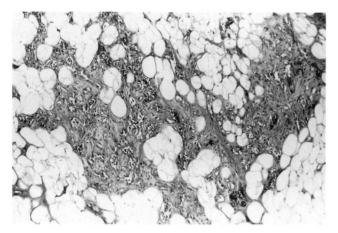

Figure 43.3. Angiolipoma.

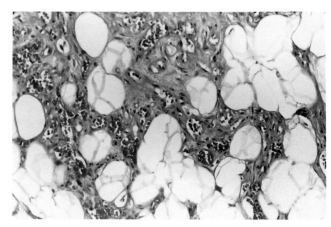

Figure 43.4. Angiolipoma.

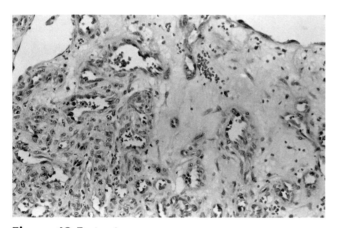

Figure 43.5. Angiosarcoma.

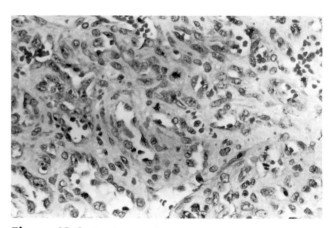

Figure 43.6. Angiosarcoma.

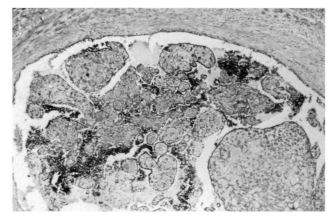

Figure 43.7. Intravascular papillary endothelial hyperplasia.

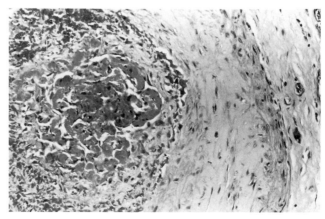

Figure 43.8. Intravascular papillary endothelial hyperplasia.

44. Poorly Differentiated Angiosarcoma vs Other Malignant Spindle Cell Tumors

Differential diagnosis of a *poorly differentiated angiosarcoma* with a predominating nonvasoformative or poorly vasoformative component (Fig. 44.1) from *other types of spindle cell sarcomas* (Fig. 44.2), *carcinomas with spindle cell metaplasia* (Fig. 44.3), and *amelanotic* *spindle cell melanomas* (Fig. 44.4) may be problematic. In these cases, the combined use of a panel of endothelial cell markers including factor VIII RA, CD31, CD34, together with EMA and anticytokeratin antibodies and HMB45, will prove helpful.

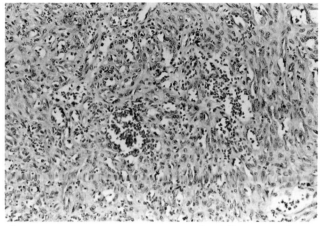

Figure 44.1. Angiosarcoma, poorly differentiated.

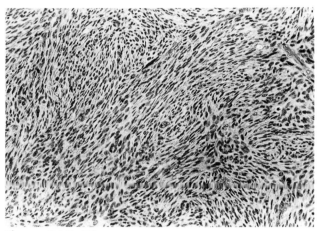

Figure 44.2. Fibrosarcoma.

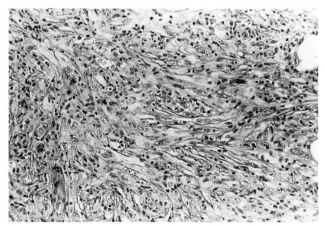

Figure 44.3. Carcinoma with prominent spindle cell metaplasia.

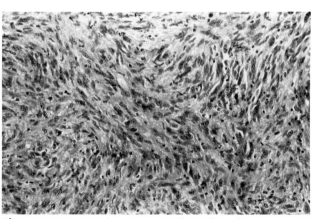

Figure 44.4. Amelanotic spindle cell melanoma.

45. Fibromatosis vs Fibrosarcoma vs Metaplastic Carcinoma

Fibromatosis is a spindle cell proliferation composed of rather uniform spindle-shaped fibroblasts with variable amounts of collagen arranged in fascicles and interlacing bundles (Figs. 45.1–45.4). This is an infiltrating lesion which entraps ducts and lobules of the breast. Focal myxoid areas may be seen. The growth patterns and the degree of cellularity of fibromatosis vary even in a single lesion. A collagenous component with an accentuated keloid-like pattern may alternate with more cellular areas. There is no cellular pleomorphism, but rare mitoses may be seen (three or four per 10 HPF). No necrosis is present. The majority of the lesions have an infiltrative periphery with stellate extensions into the adipose tissue (Figs. 45.1, 45.2, and 45.4). Ultrastructurally, a mixture of fibroblasts and myofibroblasts is seen.

Fibromatosis should be differentiated from *fibrosarcoma*. In fibrosarcoma the spindle-shaped neoplastic fibroblasts form long fascicles and herringbone patterns (Fig. 45.5). Additionally, the fibrosarcomas are usually more cellular than fibromatosis, and the cells exhibit cytologic atypia, with pleomorphism and numerous mitoses (Fig. 45.5). Areas of necrosis may also be present in fibrosarcoma.

Fibromatosis should also be differentiated from *metaplastic carcinomas* with a prominent spindle cell component (Figs. 41.3–41.6, 45.6). These tumors are usually highly cellular and may show significant pleomorphism. A carcinomatous component may be identified in metaplastic carcinomas on conventional stains if the tumor is adequately sampled (Figs. 41.3 and 41.5), and the immunoperoxidase stains for cytokeratin are of further help in demonstrating the epithelial nature, even in the apparently pure spindle cell areas (Fig. 41.6). Electron microscopy may also be helpful in making this distinction.

The absence of the characteristic cytologic and histologic features of various forms of *malignant fibrous histiocytoma* also distinguishes *fibromatosis* from this group of lesions.

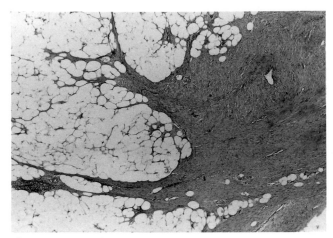

Figure 45.1. Fibromatosis.

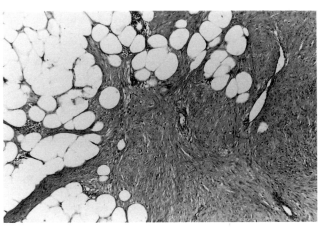

Figure 45.2. Fibromatosis.

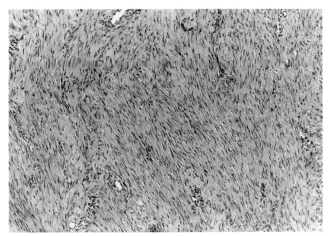

Figure 45.3. Fibromatosis.

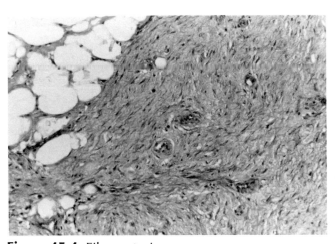

Figure 45.4. Fibromatosis.

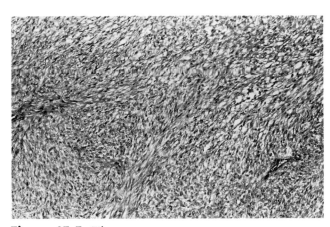

Figure 45.5. Fibrosarcoma.

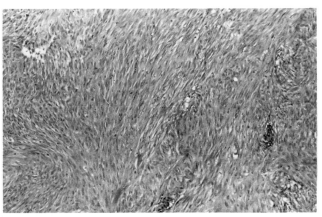

Figure 45.6. Carcinoma with prominent spindle cell metaplasia.

46. Granular Cell Tumor vs Histiocytoid Carcinoma

Granular cell tumors in the breast may histologically have a pushing or infiltrating periphery. They are composed of sheets, nests, clusters, and cords of rounded or polygonal cells with eosinophilic granular cytoplasm and round to oval, centrally located nuclei with an open chromatin pattern (Figs. 46.1–46.3). Nucleoli are often prominent, and mild nuclear pleomorphism may be present (Fig. 46.3). The cytoplasmic granules are PAS positive and diastase resistant. Nerve bundles are sometimes seen in the tumor in close association with the lesion.

When the *granular cell tumors* have an infiltrative pattern, and if there is also an associated desmoplastic reaction, the differentiation from an *infiltrating carcinoma* may sometimes be difficult. This problem is encountered specifically with the so-called *histiocytoid carcinoma*, which is considered a type of apocrine carcinoma and is also referred to as *myoblastomatoid carcinoma* by Eusebi and associates. Although some of these rare tumors show cells with foamy cytoplasm, others are composed predominantly of cells with granular cytoplasm and may sometimes be difficult to differentiate from granular cell tumors without immunohistochemistry (Figs. 46.4–46.6). Positive immunostaining reactions for cytokeratin, EMA, and gross cystic disease fluid protein-15 (GCDFP-15) (apocrine marker), together with negative staining for S-100 protein, allow an easy distinction of these carcinomas from granular cell tumors, as well as careful evaluation of the cytologic and histologic features (Figs. 46.1–46.6). In addition, if an in situ component can be demonstrated, the diagnosis of carcinoma can be easily made.

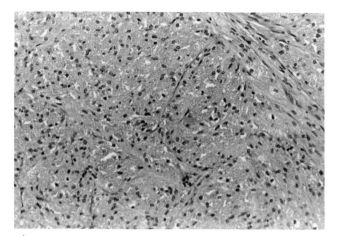

Figure 46.1. Granular cell tumor.

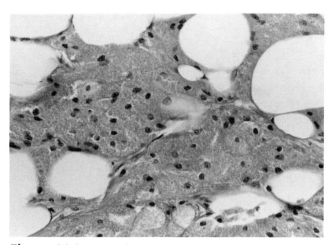

Figure 46.2. Granular cell tumor.

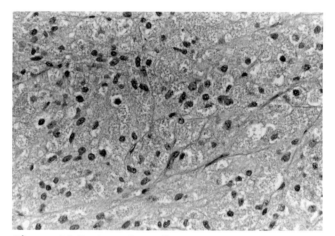

Figure 46.3. Granular cell tumor.

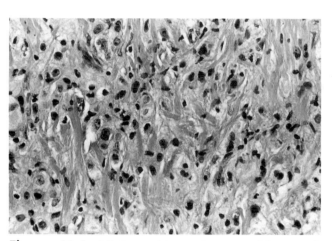

Figure 46.4. Histiocytoid carcinoma with granular cells (myoblastomatoid carcinoma).

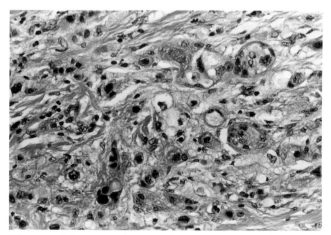

Figure 46.5. Histiocytoid carcinoma with granular cells (myoblastomatoid carcinoma).

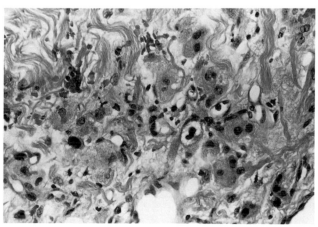

Figure 46.6. Histiocytoid carcinoma with granular cells (myoblastomatoid carcinoma).

47. Fat Necrosis vs Histiocytoid Carcinoma vs Lipid-Rich Carcinoma

Fat necrosis is histologically characterized by variably sized, lipid-filled cysts surrounded by lipid-laden histiocytes, multinucleated giant cells, and mononuclear cells intermingled with occasional clusters of neutrophils and eosinophils (Figs. 47.1 and 47.2). Fibroblastic proliferation and dense fibrosis often surround the area, and foci of calcification may also be present in this zone. Gradually, the whole area of fat necrosis is replaced by dense scar tissue.

Fat necrosis with abundant foamy histiocytes may, on rare occasions, resemble *histiocytoid carcinoma*, which is considered a type of apocrine carcinoma. As noted in Chapter 46, some of these rare tumors are composed predominantly of cells with granular cytoplasm, but others demonstrate cells with foamy cytoplasm. While the first group of lesions may resemble granular cell tumor, the second group may superficially resemble areas of fat necrosis with abundant foamy histiocytes (Figs. 47.1–47.4). In this form of histiocytoid carcinoma the cells with remarkably foamy cytoplasm show round, hyperchromatic nuclei and variable numbers of mitoses (Figs. 47.3 and 47.4). Both infiltrating lobular and ductal carcinomas are shown to be associated with this cytologic pattern. In making the distinction between *fat necrosis* with abundant foamy histiocytes and *histiocytoid carcinoma* with foamy cells, careful assessment of the overall histology is essential and immunohistochemistry is most helpful. Positive immunostaining reactions for cytokeratin, EMA, and GCDFP-15, with negative immunostaining reactions for a variety of histiocytic markers, support the diagnosis of histiocytoid carcinoma. The same markers are also helpful in differentiating histiocytoid carcinoma from xanthomatous lesions. In addition, demonstration of an in situ carcinoma component is of further help.

Lipid-rich carcinoma is composed of large cells with abundant foamy to clear cytoplasm containing neutral lipid, demonstrable with oil red O stains (Figs. 47.5 and 47.6). According to Tavassoli, lipids should be present in 80–100% of the cells for the lesion to qualify as lipid-rich carcinoma, since intracytoplasmic lipid accumulation is not uncommon in some of the other types of breast carcinoma. The tumor cells in lipid-rich carcinoma do not contain mucin or glycogen. Either DCIS or LCIS may be associated with this cytologic type of infiltrating carcinoma. Immunohistochemistry is very helpful in making the distinction between the rare *lipid-rich carcinoma* and the areas of *fat necrosis* with large numbers of foamy histiocytes. The cells of the lipid-rich carcinoma are cytokeratin and EMA positive and also stain positively for alpha lactalbumin. In areas of fat necrosis, on the other hand, various histiocyte markers are positive. Careful evaluation of the cytology and the overall histologic pattern is also essential in making this distinction (Figs. 47.1 and 47.2, 47.5 and 47.6). Demonstration of an in situ carcinoma component composed of lipid-rich cells is of additional help.

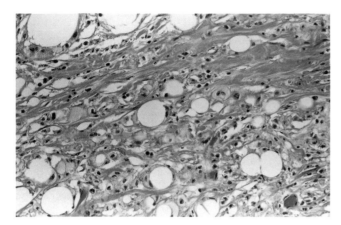

Figure 47.1. Fat necrosis.

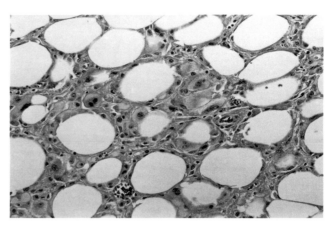

Figure 47.2. Fat necrosis.

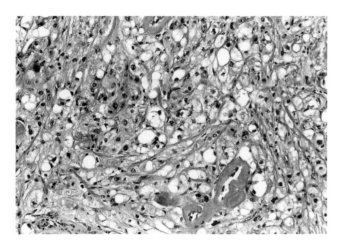

Figure 47.3. Histiocytoid carcinoma with foamy cells.

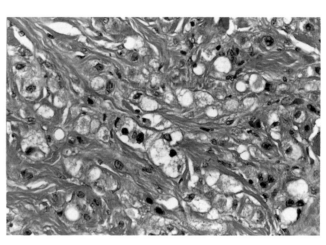

Figure 47.4. Histiocytoid carcinoma with foamy cells.

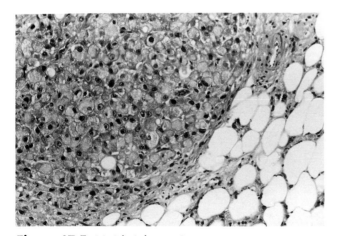

Figure 47.5. Lipid-rich carcinoma.

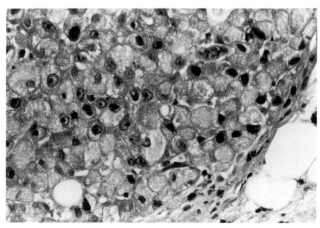

Figure 47.6. Lipid-rich carcinoma.

Section 8

LESIONS INVOLVING AXILLARY LYMPH NODES

GENERAL CONSIDERATIONS

A small group of lesions that will be discussed in this section are usually observed in resected lymph nodes, and some of them are only microscopic findings. These include reactive hyperplasia, metastatic carcinoma, lymphoma, capsular nevus cell aggregates, epithelial inclusions of skin adnexal type, and benign breast tissue inclusions. Some of these lesions, which may cause differential diagnostic problems, will be discussed in the following chapters.

48. Capsular Nevus Cell Aggregates and Nodal Glandular Inclusions vs Metastatic Tumors

Collections of cells resembling those of cutaneous nevi are sometimes found in the *capsular region of the lymph nodes.* These are most commonly seen in the axillary, inguinal, and cervical regions and only rarely in the visceral lymph nodes. They have been observed in both males and females and in all age groups. Some of these cell aggregates are found in lymph nodes of patients with malignant neoplasms such as melanoma and carcinoma, but they have also been observed in the lymph nodes of individuals with benign neoplasms and nonneoplastic conditions. Microscopically, the overall features of these cellular aggregates often mimic intradermal nevi and rarely the blue nevi. The aggregates resembling intradermal nevus cells have a band-like or nodular configuration and are located in the capsule (Figs. 48.1–48.3). They do not involve the peripheral sinuses but may extend into the lymph node along the fibrous trabeculae. Melanin pigment may be present in some of the cells. The aggregates that resemble blue nevus cells are also located in the capsule. They are composed of closely packed, heavily pigmented, spindle-shaped cells. They may extend into the surrounding perinodal adipose tissue in an irregular fashion. *Capsular nevus cell aggregates in lymph nodes* may be mistaken for *metastatic carcinoma* or melanoma, especially since the lymph node dissection usually accompanies the resection of a malignant neoplasm.

In patients with breast carcinoma, the nonpigmented cells of the *intradermal nevus type aggregates* may mimic *metastatic carcinoma,* specifically the lobular type (Fig. 48.4). They may also resemble metastatic ductal-type carcinoma, although less commonly (Figs. 48.5). The typical location of the nevus cell aggregates and the occasional presence of melanin are helpful in making this distinction, as well as the benign cytologic characteristics of the cells (Figs. 48.1–48.3). In addition, these cell aggregates are negative for mucin, show strong reactivity for S-100 protein, and are negative for cytokeratin and EMA.

In differentiating *nevus cell aggregates* from *metastatic melanoma,* their typical capsular location and bland cytologic characteristics are the most helpful features.

Other benign cellular inclusions similar to those of cutaneous eccrine and apocrine glands also occur rarely in the axillary lymph nodes (Fig. 48.6), as do the *rests of benign breast tissue,* probably representing embryonic rests. The overall benign histologic appearance of these inclusions helps in their differentiation from *metastatic adenocarcinoma.*

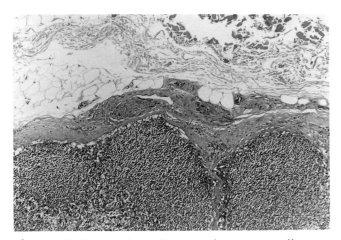

Figure 48.1. Lymph node, capsular nevus cell aggregates.

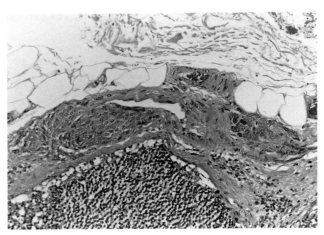

Figure 48.2. Lymph node, capsular nevus cell aggregates.

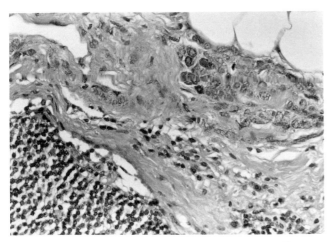

Figure 48.3. Lymph node, capsular nevus cell aggregates.

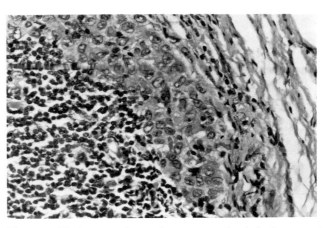

Figure 48.4. Lymph node, metastatic lobular carcinoma.

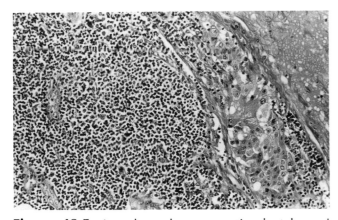

Figure 48.5. Lymph node, metastatic ductal carcinoma.

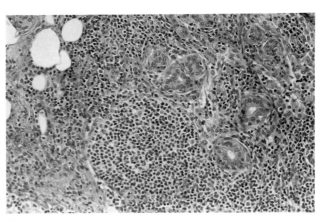

Figure 48.6. Lymph node, benign glandular inclusions.

49. Metastatic Lobular Carcinoma
vs Sinus Histiocytosis

Lymph node metastases of infiltrating *lobular carcinoma* may involve the sinusoids, and the lymphoid tissue may be largely spared in some of these cases. In such instances, distinction between the cells of the *metastatic lobular carcinoma* filling and distending the sinusoids ("sinus catarrh" pattern) (Figs. 49.1 and 49.2) from reactive histiocytes of marked *sinus histiocytosis* (Figs. 49.3 and 49.4) may be difficult. It is even more difficult to make this distinction if the reactive his-

tiocytes in sinuses demonstrate a "signet ring cell" pattern. In this rare form of sinus histiocytosis, the histiocytic cells with intracellular vacuoles may resemble the lobular carcinoma cells with intercellular lumina on hematoxylin and eosin sections, and they may also be weakly mucicarmine positive. However, the histiocytic cells are negative on immunostains for cytokeratin and EMA and are variably reactive for histiocyte markers.

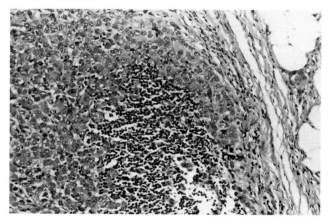

Figure 49.1. Lymph node, metastatic lobular carcinoma, "sinus catarrh" pattern.

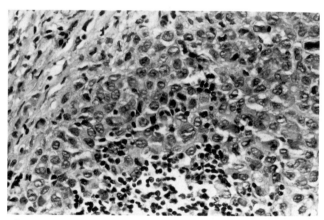

Figure 49.2. Lymph node, metastatic lobular carcinoma, "sinus catarrh" pattern.

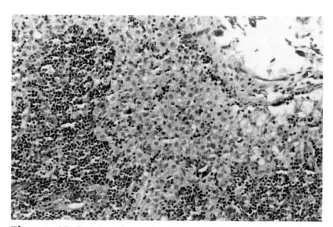

Figure 49.3. Lymph node, sinus histiocytosis.

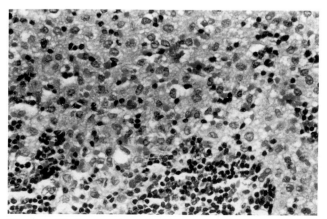

Figure 49.4. Lymph node, sinus histiocytosis.

50. Metastatic Lobular Carcinoma
vs Malignant Lymphoma

If the lymph node is diffusely replaced with *metastatic lobular carcinoma* (Fig. 50.1), its appearance may mimic that of diffuse *lymphoma* of large-cell type (Fig. 50.2). Careful assessment of the cytologic features is very important in making this distinction. In addition, mucin stains will demonstrate positivity in the region of cytoplasmic vacuoles for mucin in over 50% of the cases of metastatic lobular carcinoma. Immunohistochemical stains for cytokeratin, EMA, and LCA, along with other lymphoma-associated antigens, will prove extremely helpful in making this distinction.

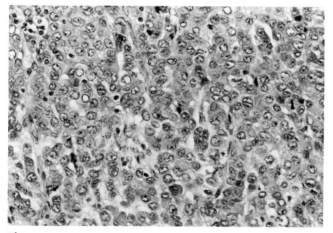

Figure 50.1. Lymph node, metastatic lobular carcinoma, diffuse pattern.

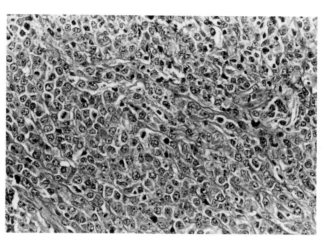

Figure 50.2. Lymph node, diffuse lymphoma, large cell type.

Section 9

SPECIMEN RADIOGRAPHS: WHAT TO LOOK FOR

GENERAL CONSIDERATIONS

Since many breast biopsies are performed for nonpalpable, mammographically detected abnormalities, it behooves the pathologist to develop some skill in recognizing such abnormalities on a specimen radiograph, whether supplied by the mammography department or obtained by an x-ray device belonging to the pathology department. Specimen radiographs are primarily done to document that the imaging abnormality that prompted the biopsy has been adequately resected. If this x-ray then accompanies the specimen to the pathol-

ogy department, it can be helpful in ensuring that the pathologist's examination is adequate. It is clearly the pathologist's duty to provide, if possible, a reasonable anatomic/pathologic correlation for the radiographically detected abnormality removed by the surgeon.

In general, imaging abnormalities that require aspiration or biopsy fall into three categories: (1) densities associated with suspicious features such as spiculated borders or distortion, (2) the development of new masses which cannot be shown to be uncomplicated cysts or fibroadenomas, and (3) calcifications which the radiologist interprets as suspicious.

51. Densities with Smooth Borders
vs Densities with Spiculation or Distortion

Most lesions which are round to oval in shape and have *smooth borders* are benign (Fig. 51.1). The majority of these are cysts, fibroadenomas, or intramammary lymph nodes, and a minority represent benign proliferative lesions such as papilloma or nodular adenosis. The radiologist may use ultrasound to distinguish cystic lesions from solid ones, and this technique sometimes reveals complex lesions with features of both, such as a papilloma within a cystically dilated duct (intracystic papilloma).

Occasionally, round or oval masses with margins which are mostly well demarcated turn out to be carcinoma. Sometimes these "round cancers" are infiltrating ductal carcinoma of no special type; however, they are likely to fulfill criteria for medullary, colloid (Fig. 51.2), or papillary carcinoma. In general, the chance of malignancy increases in a round or oval lesion as the margin becomes more obscured or ill defined.

Much more ominous radiographically are those *densities with margins which appear irregular, lobulated, or spiculated* (Fig. 51.3). Spiculated masses are usually infiltrating carcinoma (Figs. 51.4 and 51.5). However, radial sclerosing lesions may be impossible to distinguish radiologically or grossly from infiltrating carcinoma (Fig. 51.6).

Breast tissue which is biopsied for radiographic asymmetry or distortion may fail to demonstrate either carcinoma or characteristic radial scar lesions. In such cases, it is helpful for the pathologist to become more attuned to subtle changes of tissue *distortion* that might otherwise be overlooked in the search for pathologically more significant lesions. These areas of subtle distortion may represent postinflammatory periductal fibrosis related to healed periductal mastitis in duct ectasia, or to areas of irregular scarring or fibrosis of unknown etiology. The pathologist must be alert for the very subtle distortion caused by invasive lobular carcinoma and the paucity of cells that may be present in a small biopsy, particularly needle core biopsies in lobular carcinoma.

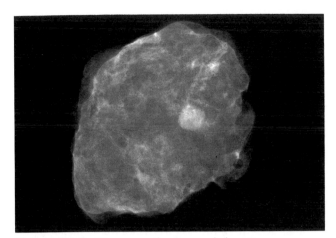

Figure 51.1. Circumscribed round density.

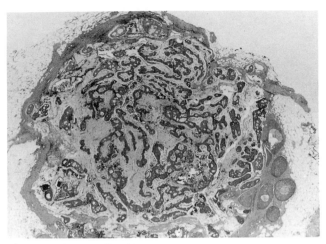

Figure 51.2. Colloid carcinoma.

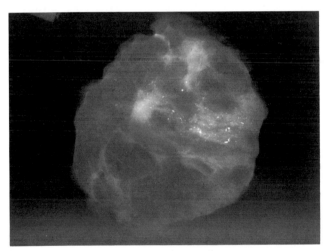

Figure 51.3. Spiculated density, linear calcifications.

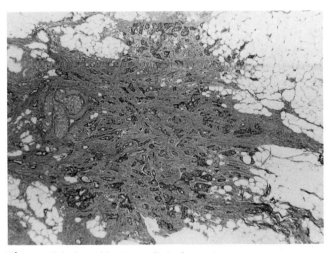

Figure 51.4. Infiltrating ductal carcinoma.

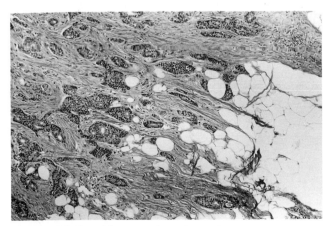

Figure 51.5. Infiltrating ductal carcinoma.

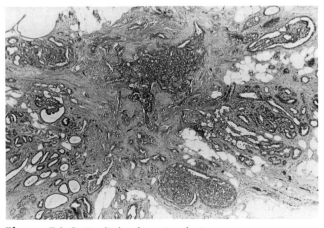

Figure 51.6. Radial sclerosing lesion.

52. Highly Suspicious Calcifications vs Calcifications of Intermediate Concern

Pathologists generally do not see many of the very benign-appearing calcifications that occur in breast tissue because these calcifications are usually not removed. These benign calcifications include the large, lobulated "popcorn" calcifications seen in sclerosed fibroadenomas and the common rod-like calcifications that occur in duct ectasia.

Calcifications which the radiologist designates as *highly suspicious*, or of *intermediate concern*, or unstable commonly come to biopsy. It then becomes the pathologist's responsibility to demonstrate these calcifications on hematoxylin and eosin sections. It is necessary that the pathologist examine the specimen radiograph, particularly in regard to the location and extent of the calcifications, and thus determine whether they are adequately represented in the histologic sections. If corresponding calcifications are not demonstrated histologically, the pathologist examines the slides under polarized light to detect calcium oxalate crystals (Figs. 52.1 and 52.2). If adequate tissue calcifications are still not identified, the pathologist requests the mammography section to x-ray the blocks to determine their locations.

Pathologists do not have the training and experience to distinguish the subtle characteristics of calcifications; however, understanding of a few basic principles may improve the accuracy of diagnostic biopsy interpreta-tion. The *most suspicious calcifications* are those which are clustered in a linear or branching fashion and appear to form a cast of the duct lumen (Figs. 51.3 and 52.3). These linear casting calcifications usually correspond to the calcifications which develop in the necrotic debris that fills the ducts in DCIS of the comedo type (Figs. 52.3–52.8).

Smaller clustered calcifications that correspond to the shape of one or more TDLUs are more problematic and may be characterized as calcifications of *indeterminate* or *intermediate concern*. Clustered, punctate calcifications that vary in size and shape may represent ductal hyperplasia or low-grade DCIS (Figs. 52.9–52.11) or, less commonly, adenosis (Fig. 52.12). Clustered, small, round calcifications which are very numerous commonly occur in association with adenosis and sclerosing adenosis (Figs. 52.13–52.16). In adenosis the calcifications usually take the shape of the small, round ductules within the affected TDLUs.

Although calcifications which develop in the aging fibroadenoma commonly have large, irregular shapes that are of no clinical concern when they are imaged, the earlier-stage small calcification in a fibroadenoma may appear clustered and indeterminate (Figs. 52.17 and 52.18) and may therefore prompt a core biopsy or excision.

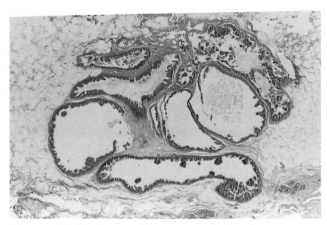

Figure 52.1. Clustered cysts, unpolarized.

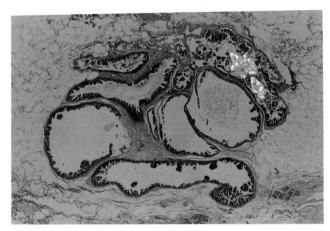

Figure 52.2. Clustered cysts with calcium oxylate crystals, polarized.

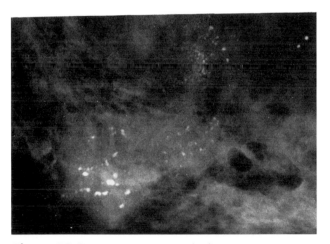

Figure 52.3. Linear, casting calcifications.

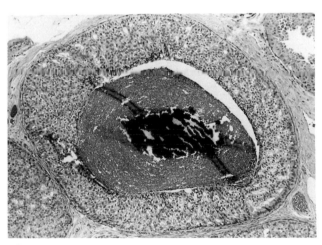

Figure 52.4. Ductal carcinoma in situ, comedo type with calcification.

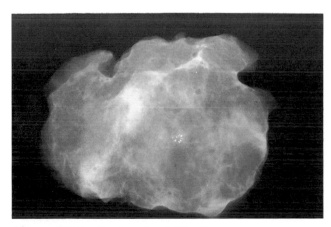

Figure 52.5. Clustered calcifications.

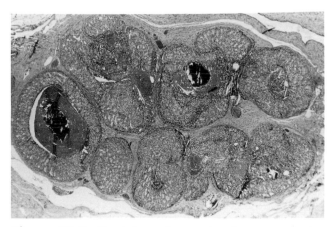

Figure 52.6. Ductal carcinoma in situ, comedo type (same case as Fig. 52.5).

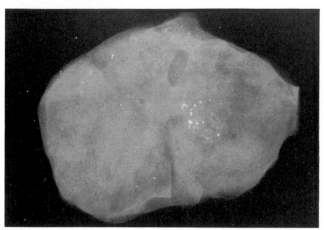

Figure 52.7. Magnified radiograph: linear calcifications.

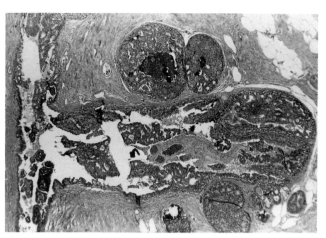

Figure 52.8. Ductal carcinoma in situ, with central necrosis and calcification.

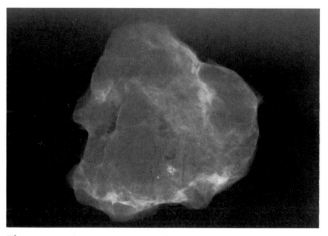

Figure 52.9. Clustered calcifications.

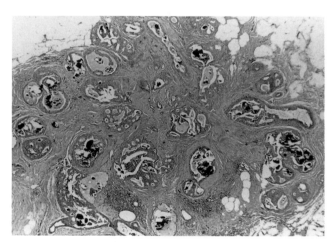

Figure 52.10. Ductal carcinoma in situ, cribriform type (same case as Fig. 52.9).

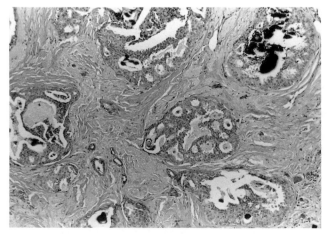

Figure 52.11. Ductal carcinoma in situ, cribriform type, intermediate grade.

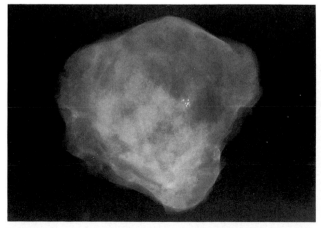

Figure 52.12. Clustered calcifications (histologically adenosis).

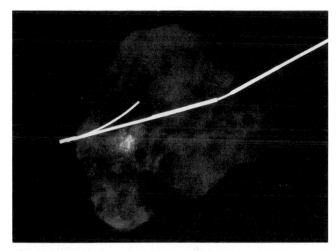

Figure 52.13. Clustered calcifications (histologically adenosis).

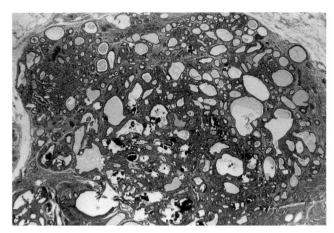

Figure 52.14. Adenosis with calcification.

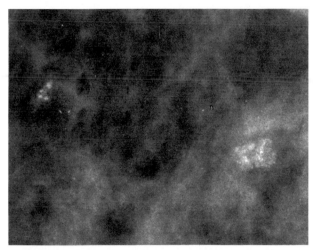

Figure 52.15. Clustered calcifications (histologically adenosis).

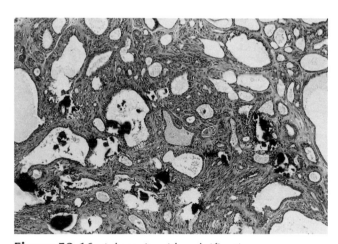

Figure 52.16. Adenosis with calcifications.

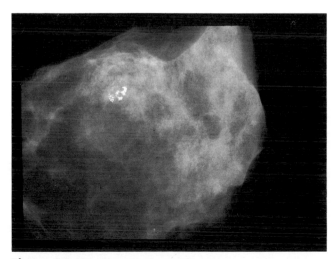

Figure 52.17. Clustered calcifications.

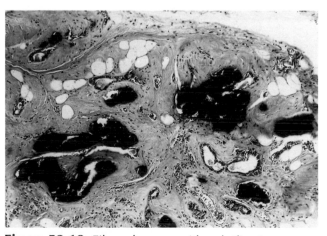

Figure 52.18. Fibroadenoma with calcification.

Section

BIBLIOGRAPHY AND INDEX

Bibliography

Section 1

Azzopardi JG: Problems in breast pathology. In Bennington JL (series ed): Major Problems in Pathology, Vol 11. Philadelphia, WB Saunders, 1979, pp 168–174.

Becker RL, Mikel UV, O'Leary TJ: Morphometric distinction of sclerosing adenosis from tubular carcinoma of the breast. *Path Res Pract* 1988:847–851, 1992.

Carter D: Interpretation of Breast Biopsies—Biopsy Interpretation Series. New York, Raven Press, 1984, pp 97–110

Carter DJ, Rosen PP: Atypical apocrine metaplasia in sclerosing lesions of the breast: A study of 51 patients. *Mod Pathol* 4:1–5, 1991.

Chan JCK, Nig WF: Sclerosing adenosis cancerized by intraductal carcinoma. *Pathology* 19:425–428, 1987.

Clement PB, Azzopardi JG: Microglandular adenosis of the breast—a lesion simulating tubular carcinoma. *Histopathology* 7:169–180, 1983.

Davies JD: Neural invasion in benign mammary dysplasia. *J Pathol* 109:225–231, 1973.

Diaz NM, McDivitt RW, Wick WR: Microglandular adenosis of the breast. An immunohistochemical comparison with tubular carcinoma. *Arch Pathol Lab Med* 115:578–582, 1991.

Eusebi V, Casadei GP, Bussolati G, et al: Adenomyoepithelioma of the breast with a distinctive type of apocrine adenosis. *Histopathology* 11:305–315, 1987.

Eusebi V, Foschini MP, Betts CM, et al: Microglandular adenosis, apocrine adenosis, and tubular carcinoma of the breast. An immunohistochemical comparison. *J Surg Pathol* 17:99–109, 1993.

Fechner RE: Lobular carcinoma in-situ in sclerosing adenosis. A potential source of confusion with invasive carcinoma. *Am J Surg Pathol* 5:233–239, 1981.

Gould VE, Rogers DR, Sommers SC: Epithelial-nerve intermingling in benign breast lesions. *Arch Pathol* 99:596–598, 1975.

Jensen PA, Page DL, Dupont WD, et al: Invasive breast cancer risk in women with sclerosing adenosis. *Cancer* 64:1977–1983, 1989.

Kay S: Microglandular adenosis of the female mammary gland: Study of a case with ultrastructural observations. *Hum Pathol* 16:637–640, 1985.

Kiaer H, Nielsen B, Paulsen S, et al: Adenomyoepithelial adenosis and low-grade malignant adenomyoepithelioma of the breast. *Virchows Arch (A)* 405:55–67, 1984.

McErlean DP, Nathan BE: Calcification in sclerosing adenosis simulating malignant breast calcification. *Br J Radiol* 45:944–945, 1972.

Nielsen BB: Adenosis tumor of the breast: A clinicopathological investigation of 27 cases. *Histopathology* 11:1259–1275, 1987.

Oberman HA: Benign breast lesions confused with carcinoma. In McDivitt RW, Oberman HA, Ozello L, et al (eds): The Breast. Baltimore, Williams & Wilkins, 1984, pp 1–33.

O'Malley FP, Page DL, Nelson EH, et al: Ductal carcinoma in-situ of the breast with apocrine cytology: Definition of a borderline category. *Hum Pathol* 25:164–168, 1994.

Page DL, Anderson TJ: Diagnostic Histopathology of the Breast. New York, Churchill Livingstone, 1987, pp 51–61.

Powell DE, Stelling CB: The Diagnosis and Detection of Breast Disease. St Louis, Mosby-Year Book, 1994, pp 261–269.

Raju U, Zarbo RJ, Kubus J, et al: The histologic spectrum of apocrine breast proliferations. *Hum Pathol* 24:173–181, 1993.

Rosen PP: Microglandular adenosis. A benign lesion simulating invasive mammary carcinoma. *Am J Surg Pathol* 7:137–144, 1983.

Rosen PP, Oberman HA: Tumors of the mammary gland. In Atlas of Tumor Pathology. Armed Forces Institute of Pathology. Washington, DC, 1993, pp 50–58.

Rosenblum MK, Purrazella R, Rosen PP: Is microglandular adenosis a precancerous disease? A study of carcinoma arising therein. *Am J Surg Pathol* 10:237–245, 1986.

Simpson JF, Page DL, Dupont MD: Aporine adenosis—a mimic of mammary carcinoma. *Surg Pathol* 3:289–299, 1990.

Tavassoli FA: Pathology of the Breast. Norwalk, CT, Appleton & Lange 1992, pp 91–107.

Tavassoli FA, Norris HJ: Microglandular adenosis of the breast. A clinicopathologic study of 11 cases with ultrastructural observations. *Am J Surg Pathol* 7:731–737, 1983.

Tavassoli FS, Norris HJ: Intraductal apocrine carcinoma. A clinicopathologic study of 37 cases. *Mod Pathol* 7:813–817, 1994.

Taylor HB, Norris HJ: Epithelial invasion of nerves in benign diseases of the breast. *Cancer* 20:2245–2249, 1967.

Wilson M, Cranor ML, Rosen PP: Papillary duct hyperplasia of the breast in children and young women. *Mod Pathol* 6:570–574, 1993.

Section 2

Anderson JA, Vendelboe ML: Cytoplasmic mucous globules in lobular carcinoma in-situ. *Am J Surg Pathol* 5:251–255, 1981.

Bellamy COC, McDonald C, Salter DM, et al: Noninvasive ductal carcinoma of the breast. The relevance of histologic categorization. *Hum Pathol* 24:16–23, 1993.

Carter DJ, Rosen PP: Atypical apocrine metaplasia in sclerosing lesions of the breast: A study of 51 patients. *Mod Pathol* 4:1–5, 1991.

Clement PB, Young RH, Azzopardi JG: Collagenous spherulosis of the breast. *Am J Surg Pathol* 11:411–417, 1987.

Dupont WD, Page DL: Risk factors for breast cancer in women with proliferative breast disease. *N Engl J Med* 312:146–151, 1985.

Dupont WD, Parl FE, Hartman WH, et al: Breast cancer risk

associated with proliferative breast disease and atypical hyperplasia. *Cancer* 71:1258–1265, 1993.

Gad A, Azzopardi JG: Lobular carcinoma of the breast: A special variant of mucin-secreting carcinoma. *J Clin Pathol* 28:711–716, 1975.

Grignon DJ, Ro JY, Mackey BN, et al: Collagenous spherulosis of the breast. Immunohistochemical and ultrastructural studies. *Am J Clin Pathol* 91:386–392, 1989.

Holland R, Hendricks JHCL: Microcalcifications associated with ductal carcinoma in-situ. Mammographic–pathologic correlation. *Semin Diagn Pathol* 11:181–192, 1994.

Holland R, Peterse JL, Mills RR, et al: Ductal carcinoma in-situ: A proposal for a new classification. *Semin Diagn Pathol* 11:167–180, 1994.

Holland R, Urbain JGM, VanHaelst, JGM: Mammary carcinoma with osteoclast-like giant cells. *Cancer* 53:1963–1973, 1984.

Lagios MD, Margolin FR, Westdahl PR, et al: Mammographically detected duct carcinoma in-situ. *Cancer* 63:618–624, 1989.

Michal M, Skalova A: Collagenous spherulosis. A comment on its histogenesis. *Path Res Pract* 1986:365–370, 1990.

O'Malley FP, Page DL, Nelson EH, et al: Ductal carcinoma in-situ of the breast with apocrine cytology. *Hum Pathol* 25:164–168, 1994.

Page DL, Anderson TJ: Diagnostic Histopathology of the Breast. New York, Churchill Livingstone, 1987, 120–191.

Page DL, Dixon JM, Anderson TJ: Invasive cribriform carcinoma of the breast. *Histopathology* 7:525–536, 1983.

Page DL, Dupont WD, Rogers LW, et al: Atypical hyperplastic lesions of the female breast. A long term follow-up study. *Cancer* 55:2698–2708, 1985.

Page DL, Kidd TE, Dupont WD, et al: Lobular neoplasia of the breast: Higher risk of subsequent invasive cancer predicted by more extensive disease. *Hum Pathol* 22:1232–1239, 1991.

Page DL, Rogers LW: Combined histologic and cytologic criteria for the diagnosis of mammary atypical ductal hyperplasia. *Hum Pathol* 23:1095–1097, 1992.

Patchefsky AS, Schwartz GF, Finkelstein SD, et al: Heterogeneity of intraductal carcinoma of the breast. *Cancer* 63:731–741, 1989.

Rosen PP, Oberman HA: Tumors of the mammary gland. In: Atlas of Tumor Pathology. Armed Forces Institute of Pathology. Washington, DC, 1993, pp 119–155.

Tavassoli FA: Pathology of the Breast. Norwalk, CT, Appleton & Lange, 1992, pp 155–191, 229–291.

Tavassoli FA, Norris HJ: A comparison of the results of long-term follow-up for atypical intraductal hyperplasia of the breast. *Cancer* 65:518–529, 1990.

Tavassoli FA, Norris HJ: Intraductal apocrine carcinoma: A clinicopathologic study of 37 cases. *Mod Pathol* 7:813–818, 1994.

Venable JG, Schwartz AM, Silverberg SG: Infiltrating cribriform carcinoma of the breast: A distinctive clinicopathologic entity. *Hum Pathol* 21:333–338, 1990.

Section 3

Azzopardi JG: Problems in Breast Pathology. Philadelphia, WB Saunders, 1979, pp 174–188.

Fenoglio C, Lattes R: Sclerosing papillary proliferations in the female breast. A benign lesion often mistaken for carcinoma. *Cancer* 33:691–700, 1974.

Page DL, Anderson TJ: Diagnostic Histopathology of the Breast. New York, Churchill Livingstone, 1987, pp. 89–103.

Nielsen M, Christensen L, Anderson J: Radial scars in women with breast cancer. *Cancer* 59:1019–1025, 1987.

Rosen pp. Oberman HA: Tumors of the Mammary Gland. In: Atlas of Tumor Pathology. Armed Forces Institute of Pathology. Washington, DC, 1993, pp 59–63.

Tavassoli FA: Pathology of the Breast. Norwalk, CT, Appleton & Lange, 1992, pp 107–114.

Tavassoli FA, Pestzner JP: Pseudoinvasion in intraductal carcinoma. *Mod Pathol* 8:380–383, 1995.

Youngson BJ, Cranor M, Rosen PP: Epithelial displacement in surgical breast specimens following needling procedures. *Am J Surg Pathol* 18:896–903, 1994.

Section 4

Azzopardi JG: Problems in breast pathology. In: Bennington, JL (series ed): Major Problems in Pathology, Vol 11. Philadelphia, WB Saunder, 1979, pp 150–166.

Azzopardi JG, Salm R: Ductal adenoma of the breast: A lesion which can mimic carcinoma. *J Pathol* 144:11–23, 1984.

Carter D: Intraductal papillary tumors of the breast. A study of 78 cases. *Cancer* 39:1689–1692, 1977.

Carter D: Interpretation of Breast Biopsies—Biopsy Interpretation Series. New York, Raven Press, 1984, pp 55–65.

Carter D, Orr SL, Merino MJ: Intracystic papillary carcinoma of the breast. After mastectomy, radiotherapy or excisional biopsy alone. *Cancer* 52:14–19, 1983.

Chan JKC, Saw D: One or two cell types in papillary carcinoma of the breast. *Pathology* 18:479–481, 1986.

Fenoglio C, Lattes R: Sclerosing papillary proliferations in the female breast. *Cancer* 33:691–700, 1974.

Flint A, Oberman HA: Infarction and squamous metaplasia of intraductal papilloma. A benign breast lesion that may simulate carcinoma. *Hum Pathol* 15:764–767, 1984.

Guarino DR, Reale D, Squilaci S, et al: Ductal adenoma of the breast. An immunohistochemical study of five cases. *Path Res Pract* 189:515–520, 1993.

Gusterson BA, Sloane JP, Middwood C, et al: Ductal adenoma of the breast—a lesion exhibiting a myoepithelial/epithelial phenotype. *Histopathology* 11:103–110, 1987.

Haagensen CD: Diseases of the Breast, ed 3. Philadelphia, WB Saunders, 1986, pp 136–174, 729–757.

Lammie GA, Millis RR: Ductal adenoma of the breast. A review of fifteen cases. *Hum Pathol* 20:903–908, 1989.

Murad TM, Contesso G, Mouriesse H: Papillary tumors of large lactiferous ducts. *Cancer* 48:122–133, 1981.

Oberman HA: Benign breast lesions confused with carcinoma. In McDivitt RW, Oberman HA, Ozello L, et al (eds): The Breast. Baltimore: Williams & Wilkins, 1984, pp 1–33.

Page DL, Anderson TJ: Diagnostic Histopathology of the Breast. Edinburgh, Churchill Livingstone, 1987, pp 104–119, 186–190.

Page DL, Zwang RV, Rogers LW, et al: Relation between component parts of fibrocystic disease complex and breast cancer. *J Natl Cancer Instit* 61:1055–1063, 1978.

Papotti M, Gugliotta P, Eusebi V, et al: Immunohistochemical analysis of benign and malignant papillary lesions of the breast. *Am J Surg Pathol* 7:451–461, 1983.

Papotti M. Gugliotta P, Ghiringihello B, et al: Association of breast carcinoma and multiple intraductal papillomas: A histological and immunohistochemical investigation. *Histopathology* 8:963–975, 1984.

Powell DE, Stelling CB: The Diagnosis and Detection of Breast Disease. St Louis, Mosby-Year Book, 1994, pp 192–204.

Ramos CV, Boeshart C, Restrapo GL: Intracystic papillary carcinoma of the male breast. *Arch Pathol Lab Med* 109: 858–861, 1985.

Rosen PP, Oberman HA: Tumors of the mammary gland. In Atlas of Tumor Pathology. Armed Forces Institute of Pathology. Washington, DC, 1993, pp 72–78, 209–218.

Tavassoli FA: Pathology of the Breast. Norwalk, CT, Appleton & Lange 1992, pp 193–228.

Tavassoli FA, Norris HJ: Intraductal apocrine carcinoma. A clinical study of 37 cases. *Mod Pathol* 7:813–817, 1994.

Wilson M, Cranor ML, Rosen PP: Papillary duct hyperplasia of the breast in children and young women. *Mod Pathol* 6:570–574, 1993.

Section 5

Cohen PL, Brooks JJ: Lymphomas of the breast. A clinicopathologic and immunohistochemical study of primary and secondary cases. *Cancer* 67:1359–1369, 1991.

DiCostanzo P, Rosen PP, Garren I et al: Prognosis in infiltrating lobular carcinoma. An analysis of "classical" and variant tumors. *Am J Surg Pathol* 14:12–23, 1990.

Dixon JM, Anderson JJ, Page DL et al: Infiltrating lobular carcinoma of the breast. *Histopathology* 6:149–161, 1982.

Eusebi V, Magalhaes F, Azzopardi JG et al: Pleomorphic lobular carcinoma of the breast. An aggressive tumor showing apocrine differentiation. *Hum Pathol* 23:655–662, 1992.

Fechner RE: Histologic variants of infiltrating lobular carcinoma of the breast. *Hum Pathol* 6:373–378, 1975.

Fischer ER, Gregorio RM, Redmond C et al: Tubulolobular invasive breast cancer. A variant of lobular invasive cancer. *Hum Pathol* 8:679–683, 1977.

Holland R, vanHaelst UJ: Mammary carcinoma with osteoclast-like giant cells. *Cancer* 53:1963–1973, 1984.

Hugh JC, Jackson FI, Hanson J et al: Primary breast lymphoma. *Cancer* 66:2602–2611, 1990.

Kaufman MW, Marti JR, Gallager HS et al: Carcinoma of the breast with pseudosarcomatous metaplasia. *Cancer* 53: 1908–1917, 1984.

Martinez V, Azzopardi JG: Invasive lobular carcinoma of the breast. Incidence and variants. *Histopathology* 3:467–488, 1979.

Oberman HA: Metaplastic carcinoma of the breast. A clinicopathologic study of 29 patients. *Am J Surg Pathol* 11:918–929, 1987.

Page DL, Anderson JJ: Diagnostic Histopathology of the Breast. New York, Churchill Livingstone, 1987, pp 210–215.

Page DL, Dixon JM, Anderson TJ et al: Invasive cribriform carcinoma of the breast. *Histopathology* 7:525–536, 1983.

Parl FF, Richardson LD: The histological and biological spectrum of tubular carcinoma of the breast. *Hum Pathol* 14:694–698, 1983.

Rapin V, Contesso G, Mouriesse H et al: Medullary breast carcinoma: A revaluation of 95 cases of breast cancer with inflammatory stroma. *Cancer* 61:2503–2510, 1988.

Ridolfi RE, Rosen PP, Port A et al: Medullary carcinoma of the breast: A clinical pathological study with 10 years follow-up. *Cancer* 40:1365–1385, 1977.

Ro JY, Sneige N, Sahin AA et al: Mucocele-like tumor of the breast with atypical ductal hyperplasia or mucinous carcinoma. *Arch Pathol Lab Med* 115:137–140, 1991.

Rosen PP: Mucocele-like tumors of the breast. *Am J Surg Pathol* 10:464–469, 1986.

Rosen PP, Cantrell B, Mullen DL et al: Juvenile papillomatosis (Swiss cheese disease) of the breast. *Am J Surg Pathol* 4:3–12, 1980.

Rosen PP, Ernsberger D: Low-grade adenosquamous carcinoma. A variant of metaplastic mammary carcinoma. *Am J Surg Pathol* 11:351–358, 1987.

Rosen PP, Oberman HA: Tumors of the Mammary Gland, In Atlas of Tumor Pathology. Armed Forces Institute of Pathology. Washington, DC, 1993, pp 182–186, 187–193, 194–206, 226–231.

Rosen PP, Scott M: Cystic hypersecretory duct carcinoma of the breast. *Am J Surg Pathol* 8:31–41, 1984.

Tavassoli FA: Pathology of the Breast. Norwalk, CT, Appleton and Lange, 1992, pp 315–320, 320–325, 333–339, 403–414, 624–630.

Tavassoli FA: Classification of metaplastic carcinomas of the breast. In Rosen PP, Fecher RD (eds), Pathology Annual, Vol 27. Norwalk, CT, Appleton and Lange, 1992, 89–119.

Venable JG, Schwartz AM, Silverberg SG et al: Infiltrating cribriform carcinoma of the breast. A distinctive clinicopathologic entity. *Hum Pathol* 21:333–338, 1990.

Wargotz ES, Deos PH, Norris HJ et al: Metaplastic carcinomas of the breast. II. Spindle cell carcinoma. *Hum Pathol* 21:732–740, 1989.

Wargotz ES, Norris HJ: Metaplastic carcinomas of the breast. I. Matrix-producing carcinoma. *Hum Pathol* 20:628–635, 1989.

Wargotz ES, Norris HJ: Metaplastic carcinoma of the breast. IV. Squamous cell carcinoma of ductal origin. *Cancer* 65:272–276, 1990.

Weaver MG, Abdul-Karim FW, Al-Kaisi N et al: Mucinous lesions for the breast: A pathological continuum. *Pathol Res Pract* 189:873–876, 1993.

Weidner N, Semple JP: Pleomorphic variant of invasive lobular carcinoma of the breast. *Hum Pathol* 23:1167–1171, 1992.

Section 6

Gillett CE, Bobrow LG, Millis RR et al: S-100 protein in human mammary tissue—immunoreactivity in breast carcinoma, including Paget disease of the nipple. *J Pathol* 160:19–24, 1990.

Rosen PP: Syringomatous adenoma of the nipple. *Am J Surg Pathol* 7:739–745, 1983

Rosen PP, Caicco JA: Florid papillomatosis of the nipple: A study of 51 patients including nine with mammary carcinoma. *Am J Surg Pathol* 10:87–101, 1986.

Rosen PP, Oberman HA: Florid papillomatosis of the nipple. In Tumors of the Mammary Gland. Washington, DC, Armed Forces Institute of Pathology, 1993, pp 78–87.

Rosen PP, Oberman HA: Tumors of the Mammary Gland. In Atlas of Tumor Pathology. Armed Forces Institute of Pathology. Washington, DC, 1993, pp 266–270.

Tavassoli, FA: Pathology of the Breast. Norwalk, CT, Appleton and Lange, 1992, pp 583–589.

Section 7

Altavilla G, Cavazzini L, Rossi S: Osteogenic sarcoma of the breast. A case report and review of the literature. Pathologica 77:101–106, 1985.

Austin RM, Dupree WB: Liposarcoma of the breast: A clinicopathologic study of 20 cases. *Hum Pathol* 17:906–913, 1986.

Azzopardi JG: Problems in breast pathology. In Bennington, JL (series ed): Major Problems in Pathology, Vol. 11. Philadelphia, WB Saunders, 1979, pp 39–56, 253–254, 297–302, 354–355, 368–371.

Barnes L, Pietruszka M: Sarcomas of the breast. A clinicopathologic analysis of ten cases. *Cancer* 40:1577–1585, 1977.

Barnes L, Pietruszka M: Rhabdomyosarcoma arising within a cystosarcoma phyllodes. Case report and review of the literature. *Am J Surg Pathol* 2:423–429, 1978.

Berean K, Tron VA, Churg A, et al: Mammary fibroadenoma with multinucleated stromal giant cells. *Am J Surg Pathol* 10:823–827, 1986.

Berg JW, DeCosse JJ, Fracchia AA, et al: Stromal sarcoma of the breast. A unified approach to connective tissue sarcomas other than cystosarcoma phyllodes. *Cancer* 15:418–424, 1962.

Carney JA, Gordon H, Carpenter PC, et al: The complex of myxomas, spotty pigmentation, and endocrine overactivity. *Medicine* 64:270–283, 1985.

Carney JA, Toorkey BC: Myxoid fibroadenoma and allied conditions (myxomatosis) of the breast. A heritable disorder with special associations including cardial and cutaneous myxomas. *Am J Surg Pathol* 15:713–721, 1991.

Carstens PHB, Cooke JL: Mammary carcinosarcoma presenting as rhabdomyosarcoma. An ultrastructural and immunocytochemical study. *Ultrastruct Pathol* 14:537–544, 1990.

Chen KTK: Rare variants of benign vascular tumors of the breast. *Surg Pathol* 4:309–316, 1991.

Costa J, Wesley RA, Glatstein E, et al: The grading of soft tissue sarcomas. Results of a clinicopathologic correlation in a series of 163 cases. *Cancer* 53:530–541, 1984.

Demay RM, Kay S: Granular cell tumor of the breast. *Pathol Annu* 19:121–148, 1984.

Diaz NM, Palmer JO, McDivitt RW: Carcinoma arising within fibroadenomas of the breast. A clinicopathologic study of 105 patients. *Am J Clin Pathol* 95:614–622, 1991.

Donnell RM, Rosen PP, Lieberman PH, et al: Angiosarcoma and other vascular tumors of the breast: Pathologic analysis as a guide to prognosis. *Am J Surg Pathol* 5:629–642, 1981.

Dupont WD, Page DL, Parl FF, et al: Long-term risk of breast cancer in women with fibroadenoma. *N Engl J Med* 331:10–15, 1994.

Elhence IP, Mital VP, Upadhayaya SC, et al: Rhabdomyosarcoma of breast. *Ind J Cancer* 9:171–174, 1972.

El-Naggar AK, Ro JY, McLemore D, et al: DNA content and proliferative activity of cystosarcoma phyllodes of the breast: Potential prognostic significance. *Am J Clin Pathol* 93:980–985, 1990.

Enzinger FM, Weiss SW: Soft Tissue Pathology. St Louis, Mosby, 1995.

Eusebi V, Foschini MP, Bussolati G, et al: Myoblastomatoid (histiocytoid) carcinoma of the breast. A type of apocrine carcinoma. *Am J Surg Pathol* 19:553–562, 1995.

Fekete P, Petrek J, Majmudar B, et al: Fibroadenomas with stromal cellularity. A clinicopathologic study of 21 patients. *Arch Pathol Lab Med* 111:427–432, 1987.

Going JJ, Lumsden AB, Anderson TJ: A classical osteogenic sarcoma of the breast: Histology, immunohistochemistry and ultrastructure. *Histopathology* 10:631–641, 1986.

Grimes MM: Cystosarcoma phyllodes of the breast: Histologic features, flow cytometric analysis, and clinical correlations. *Mod Pathol* 5:232–239, 1992.

Haggitt RC, Booth JI: Bilateral fibromatosis for the breast in Gardner's syndrome. *Cancer* 25:161–166, 1970.

Harris M, Persaud V: Carcinosarcoma of the breast. *J Pathol* 112:99–105, 1974.

Hart WR, Bauer RC, Oberman HA: Cystosarcoma phyllodes. A clinicopathologic study of twenty-six hypercellular periductal stromal tumors of the breast. *Am J Clin Pathol* 70:211–216, 1978.

Hawkins RE, Schofield JB, Fisher C, et al: The clinical and histologic criteria that predicts metastases from cystosarcoma phyllodes. *Cancer* 69:141–147, 1992.

Hoda SA, Cranor ML, Rosen PP: Hemangiomas of the breast with atypical histological features. Further analysis of histological subtypes confirming their benign character. *Am J Surg Pathol* 16:553–560, 1992.

Ibrahim RE, Schiotto CG, Weidner N: Pseudoangiomatous hyperplasia of mammary stroma. Some observations regarding its clinicopathologic spectrum. *Cancer* 63:1154–1160, 1989.

Jozefczyk MA, Rosen PP: Vascular tumors of the breast II. Perilobular hemangiomas and hemangiomas. *Am J Surg Pathol* 9:491–503, 1985.

Kahn LB, Uys CJ, Dale J, et al: Carcinoma of the breast with metaplasia to chondrosarcoma: A light and electron microscopic study. *Histopathology* 2:93–106, 1978.

Knudsen PJT, Ostergaard J: Cystosarcoma phyllodes with lobular and ductal carcinoma in situ. *Arch Pathol Lab Med* 111:873–875, 1987.

Langham MR Jr: Malignant fibrous histiocytoma of the breast. A case report and review of the literature. *Cancer* 54:558–563, 1984.

McDivitt RW, Urban JA, Farrow JH: Cystosarcoma phyllodes. *Johns Hopkins Med J* 120:33–45, 1967.

Merino M, Carter D, Berman M: Angiosarcoma of the breast: A clinicopathologic study. *Am J Surg Pathol* 7:53–60, 1983.

Murad TM, Hines JR, Bauer J, et al: Histopathologic and clinical correlations of cystosarcoma phyllodes. *Arch Pathol Lab Med* 112:752–756, 1988.

Norris HJ, Taylor HB: Relationship of histologic features to behavior of cystosarcoma phyllodes: Analysis of ninety-four cases. *Cancer* 20:2090–2099, 1967.

Oshawa M, Naka N, Tomita Y, et al: Use of immunohistochemical procedures in diagnosing angiosarcoma. *Cancer* 75:2867–2874, 1995.

Page DL, Anderson TJ: Diagnostic Histopathology of the Breast. New York, Churchill Livingstone, 1987, pp 62–68, 72–85, 249–252, 256, 312–313, 335–353.

Palko MJ, Wang SE, Shackey SE, et al: Flow cytometric S fraction as a predictor of clinical outcome in cystosarcoma phyllodes. *Arch Pathol Lab Med* 114:949–952, 1990.

Pardo-Mindan J, Garcia-Julian G, Eizaguirre AM, et al: Leiomyosarcoma of the breast. *Am J Clin Pathol* 62:477–480, 1974.

Pietruszka M, Barnes L: Cystosarcoma phyllodes. A clinicopathologic analysis of 42 cases. *Cancer* 41:1974–1983, 1978.

Pike AM, Oberman HA: Juvenile (cellular) adenofibromas. A clinicopathologic study. *Am J Surg Pathol* 9:730–736, 1985.

Powell CM, Cranor ML, Rosen PP: Pseudoangiomatous stromal hyperplasia (PASH). A mammary stromal tumor with myofibroblastic proliferation. *Am J Surg Pathol* 19:270–277, 1995.

Powell DE, Stelling CB: The Diagnosis and Detection of Breast Disease. St Louis, Mosby, 1994, pp 159–177, 344–378.

Raju GC, O'Reilly AP: Immunohistochemical study of granular cell tumor. *Pathology* 19:402–406, 1987.

Rosen PP: Vascular tumors of the breast III. Angiomatosis. Am *J Surg Pathol* 9:652–658, 1985.

Rosen PP, Jozefczyk MA, Boram LH: Vascular tumors of the breast IV. The venous hemangioma. *Am J Surg Pathol* 9:659–665, 1985.

Rosen PP, Kimmel M, Ernsberger D: Mammary angiosarcoma. A prognostic significance of tumor differentiation. *Cancer* 62:2145–2151, 1988.

Rosen PP, Oberman HA: Tumors of the mammary gland. In Atlas of Tumor Pathology. Armed Forces Institute of Pathology. Washington, DC, 1993, pp 23, 101–114, 194–203, 242, 293–334.

Tavassoli FA: Classification of metaplastic carcinomas of the breast. In Rosen PP, Fechner RD (eds): Pathology Annual Vol 27. Norwalk CT, Appleton and Lange, 19, pp 89–119.

Tavassoli FA: Pathology of the Breast. Norwalk CT, Appleton and Lange, 1992, pp 379–381, 425–563.

Vuitch MF, Rosen PP, Erlandson RA: Pseudoangiomatous hyperplasia of mammary stroma. *Hum Pathol* 17:185–191, 1986.

Ward RM, Evans HL: Cystosarcoma phyllodes. A clinicopathologic study of 26 cases. *Cancer* 58:2282–2289, 1986.

Wargotz ES, Norris HJ: Metaplastic carcinomas of the breast III. Carcinosarcoma. *Cancer* 64:1490–1499, 1989.

World Health Organization: Histologic typing of breast tumors. In International Histological Classification of Tumors, ed 2, no 2. Geneva, World Health Organization, 1981.

Section 8

Azzopardi JG: Problems in breast pathology. In Bennington, JL (series ed): Major Problems in Pathology, Vol. 11. Philadelphia, WB Saunders, 1979, pp 316–318.

Azzopardi JG, Ross CM, Frizzera G: Blue nevi of lymph node capsule. *Histopathology* 1:451–461, 1977.

Edlow DW, Carter D: Heterotopic epithelium in axillary lymph nodes: Report of a case and review of the literature. *Am J Clin Pathol* 59:666–673, 1973.

Epstein JI, Erlandson RA, Rosen PP: Nodal blue nevi. A study of three cases. *Am J Surg Pathol* 8:907–915, 1982.

Gould E, Perez J, Albores-Saavedra J, et al: Signet ring cell sinus histiocytoses. A previously unrecognized histologic condition mimicking metastatic adenocarcinoma in the lymph nodes. *Am J Clin Pathol* 92:509–512, 1989.

Holdsworth PJ, Hopkinson JM, Leveson SH: Benign axillary

epithelial lymph node inclusions—a histological pitfall. *Histopathology* 13:266–228, 1988.

Page DL, Anderson TJ: Diagnostic Histopathology of the Breast. New York, Churchill Livingstone, 1987, p 314–329.

Ridolfi RL, Rosen PP, Thaler H: Nevus cell aggregates associated with lymph nodes: Estimated frequency and clinical significance. *Cancer* 39:164–171, 1977.

Rosen PP, Oberman HA: Tumors of the mammary gland. In Atlas of Tumor Pathology. Armed Forces Institute of Pathology, Washington, DC, 1993, pp 355–365.

Tavassoli FA: Pathology of the Breast. Norwalk, CT, Appleton and Lange, 1992, pp 304–306.

Turner DR, Millis PR: Breast tissue inclusions in axillary lymph nodes. *Histopathology* 4:631–636, 1980.

Section 9

American College of Radiology: Breast imaging reporting and data system. Reston, VA, American College of Radiology, 1993.

Bassett LW: Mammographic analysis of calcifications. *Radiol Clin North Am* 30:93–105, 1992.

Evans WP: Breast masses. *Radiol Clin North Am* 33:1085–1108, 1995.

Feig SA: Breast masses. Mammographic and sonographic evaluation. *Radiol Clin North Am* 30:67–92, 1992.

Monsees BS: Evaluation of breast microcalcifications. *Radiol Clin North Am* 33:1109–1121, 1995.

INDEX

A

Adenosis, 1–23
with calcifications, *173*
clinical overview, 1
ductal carcinoma *in situ* in sclerosing adenosis vs. infiltrating ductal carcinoma, 18–19, *19*
ductal carcinoma *in situ* in sclerosing adenosis, *19*
infiltrating ductal carcinoma, *19*
ductal hyperplasia, atypical and ductal carcinoma *in situ* in sclerosing adenosis vs. atypical lobular hyperplasia and lobular carcinoma *in situ* in sclerosing adenosis, 22–23, *23*
ductal carcinoma *in situ* in adenosis, *23*
lobular carcinoma *in situ* in adenosis, *23*
gross morphology, overview, 1
imaging, 1
lobular carcinoma *in situ* in sclerosing adenosis vs. infiltrating lobular carcinoma, 20–21, *21*
infiltrating lobular carcinoma, *21*
lobular carcinoma *in situ* in sclerosing adenosis, *21*
microglandular vs. tubular carcinoma, 14–15, *15*
microglandular adenosis, *15*
tubular carcinoma, *15*
normal lobule, *3*
overview, 1
sclerosing, *see* Sclerosing adenosis
Angiosarcoma
vs. benign vascular proliferations, 150–152, *152*
angiolipoma, *152*
angiosarcoma, *151, 152*
hemangioma, *151, 152*
Intravascular papillary endothelial hyperplasia, *152*
vs. mammary stroma, pseudoangiomatous hyperplasia of, 148–149, *149*
angiosarcoma, *149*
pseudoangiomatous hyperplasia of mammary stroma, *149*
poorly differentiated, vs. other spindle cell tumors, 153, *153*
amelanotic spindle cell melanoma, *153*
angiosarcoma, poorly differentiated, *153*
carcinoma with prominent spindle cell metaplasia, *153*
fibrosarcoma, *153*
Apocrine carcinoma vs. sclerosing adenosis, non-neoplastic apocrine alterations in, 8–11, *9, 11*
apocrine ductal carcinoma *in situ* in sclerosing adenosis, *9, 11*
apocrine hyperplasia in sclerosing adenosis, atypical, *9*
apocrine metaplasia in sclerosing adenosis, *9, 11*
apocrine metaplasia in sclerosing adenosis, atypical, *11*
infiltrating apocrine carcinoma, *11*
Apocrine hyperplasia and atypical apocrine hyperplasia vs. intraductal apocrine carcinoma, 42–45, *43, 45*
apocrine hyperplasia, *43*
apocrine ductal carcinoma *in situ*, *45*
atypical apocrine hyperplasia, *43*
papillary apocrine hyperplasia, *43*
Axillary lymph node lesions, 161–165
benign glandular inclusions, *163*
capsular nevus cell aggregates, *163*
malignant lymphoma, *165*
metastatic ductal carcinoma, *163*
metastatic lobular carcinoma, *163, 165*
sinus histiocytosis, *165*

B

Biphasic and mesenchymal proliferations, 124–159
angiosarcoma, poorly differentiated, vs. other spindle cell tumors, 153, *153*

amelanotic spindle cell melanoma, *153*
angiosarcoma, poorly differentiated, *153*
carcinoma with prominent spindle cell metaplasia, *153*
fibrosarcoma, *153*
carcinosarcoma vs. metaplastic carcinoma vs. pure sarcoma, 146–147, *147*
carcinoma with prominent spindle cell metaplasia, cytokeratin immunoperoxidase, *147*
carcinoma with prominent spindle cell metaplasia, *147*
carcinoma with spindle cell metaplasia, *147*
carcinoma with squamous and spindle cell metaplasia, *147*
metaplastic carcinoma, *147*
clinical overview, 125–126
fat necrosis vs. histiocytoid carcinoma vs. lipid-rich carcinoma, 158–159, *159*
fat necrosis, *159*
histiocytoid carcinoma with foamy cells, *159*
lipid-rich carcinoma, *159*
fibroadenoma vs. low-grade phyllodes tumor, 128–135, *130–135*
cellular fibroadenoma, *131, 135*
ductal carcinoma *in situ* in fibroadenoma, *132*
fibroadenoma
with apocrine metaplasia, *131*
with fibrocystic changes, *131*
fine needle aspiration, *130*
intracanalicular pattern, *130, 135*
mixed pattern, *130*
pericanalicular pattern, *130*
with usual epithelial hyperplasia, *131*
fibroadenoma phyllodes, *131, 135*
lobular carcinoma *in situ*
in fibroadenoma, *132*
in phyllodes tumor, *134*
phyllodes tumor, *132, 133*
core needle biopsy, *133*
with fibrocystic changes, *133*
fine needle aspiration, *133*
with liposarcomatous stroma, *134*
low grade, *135*
with spindle cell (fibrosarcomatous) stroma, *134*
fibroadenoma with superimposed sclerosing adenosis vs. fibroadenoma with infiltrating carcinoma, 138–139, *139*
adenosis in fibroadenoma, *139*
infiltrating lobular carcinoma in fibroadenoma, *139*
infiltrating tubular carcinoma in fibroadenoma, *139*
sclerosing adenosis with attenuated ductules in fibroadenoma, *139*
fibromatosis vs. fibrosarcoma vs. metaplastic carcinoma, 154–155, *155*
carcinoma with prominent spindle cell metaplasia, *155*
fibromatosis, *155*
fibrosarcoma, *155*
granular cell tumor vs. histiocytoid carcinoma, 156–157, *157*
granular cell tumor, *157*
histiocytoid carcinoma with granular cells (myoblastomatoid carcinoma), *157*
gross morphology, overview, 127
imaging, 126
juvenile fibroadenoma vs. fibroadenoma of adult type vs. low-grade phyllodes tumor, 136–137, *137*
fibroadenoma, *137*
juvenile fibroadenoma, *137*
phyllodes tumor, *137*
overview, 124–125

periductal stromal sarcoma vs. phyllodes tumor vs. pure sarcoma, 144–145, *145*
periductal stromal sarcoma, *145*
phyllodes tumor, *145*
pure spindle cell sarcoma, *145*
phyllodes tumor
high-grade, with sarcomatous overgrowth vs. pure sarcoma, 142–143, *143*
phyllodes tumor, high grade
with fibrosarcomatous stromal overgrowth, *143*
with liposarcomatous stromal overgrowth, *143*
low-grade vs. high-grade phyllodes tumor, 140–141, *141*
phyllodes tumor
high grade, *141*
low grade, *141*
pseudoangiomatous hyperplasia of mammary stroma vs. angiosarcoma, 148–149, *149*
angiosarcoma, *149*
pseudoangiomatous hyperplasia of mammary stroma, *149*
vascular proliferations, benign, vs. angiosarcoma, 150–152, *152*
angiolipoma, *151, 152*
angiosarcoma, *152*
hemangioma, *151, 152*
intravascular papillary endothelial hyperplasia, *152*

C

Calcifications, highly suspicious vs. calcifications of intermediate concern, 170–173, *171–173*
adenosis, with calcification, *173*
clustered calcification, *171–173*
clustered cysts
with calcium oxalate crystals, polarized, *171*
unpolarized, *171*
ductal carcinoma *in situ*
with central necrosis and calcification, *172*
comedo type, *171*
cribriform type, *172*
fibroadenoma with calcification, *173*
linear, casting calcifications, *171*
Carcinoma. See also ductal and lobular proliferations, papillary lesions and special types of infiltrating carcinoma
in-situ, ductal
apocrine type, vs. apocrine hyperplasia and atypical apocrine hyperplasia, 42–45, *43, 45*
arising in papilloma, vs. atypical epithelial hyperplasia in papilloma, 80, *80*
cribriform type, vs. collagenous spherulosis vs. adenoid cystic carcinoma, 52–53, *53*
cribriform type, vs. infiltrating cribriform carcinoma, 88–93, *90–93*
vs. infiltrating ductal carcinoma, in sclerosing adenosis, 18–19, *19*
vs. lobular carcinoma in situ, in sclerosing adenosis, 20–21, *21*
papillary type, with pseudoinfiltration vs. infiltrating papillary carcinoma, 80–81, *81*
vs. usual ductal hyperplasia and atypical ductal hyperplasia, 30–35, *31–35*
lobular extension of, vs. ductal extension of LCIS, 48–51, *49–51*
within radial sclerosing lesions, vs. usual radial scars and infiltrating carcinoma, 58–61, *59–61*
in-situ, lobular
vs. ductal carcinoma in situ, in sclerosing adenosis, 22–23, *23*
ductal extension of, vs. lobular extension of DCIS, 48–51, *49–51*

Carcinoma *(contd.)*
and ALH in radial sclerosing lesions vs.
infiltrating carcinoma, 62–63, *63*
vs. infiltrating lobular carcinoma, in sclerosing
adenosis, 20–21, *21*
vs. usual lobular hyperplasia and atypical
lobular hyperplasia, 46–47, *47*
infiltrating. See also special types of
vs. DCIS within radial sclerosing lesions, vs.
usual radial scars, 58–61, *59–61*
in fibroadenoma, vs. fibroadenoma with
superimposed adenosis, 138–139, *139*
histiocytoid type
vs. fat necrosis vs. lipid-rich carcinoma,
158–159, *159*
vs. granular cell tumor, 156–157, *157*
lipid-rich type
vs. fat necrosis, vs. histiocytoid carcinoma,
158–159, *159*
associated with papilloma, vs. papilloma with
sclerotic alterations, 74–75, *75*
perineural invasion in, vs. perineural space
extension in sclerosing adenosis, 6–7, *7*
vs. post biopsy and traumatic alterations in in
situ carcinoma, 64–65, *65*
vs. radial sclerosing lesions, 55–57, *56–57*
infiltrating, ductal
tubular type,
vs. sclerosing adenosis, 2–5, *3–5*
vs. microglandular adenosis, 14–15, *15*
vs. other types of infiltrating carcinoma,
84–87, *85–87*
adenoid cystic type, vs. cribriform DCIS vs.
collagenous spherulosis, 88–93, *92, 93*
apocrine type vs. nonneoplastic apocrine
alterations in sclerosing adenosis, 8–11,
9–11
vs. DCIS in sclerosing adenosis, 18–19, *19*
cribriform type, vs. cribriform DCIS, 40–41,
41
cribriform type, vs. ductal DCIS of cribriform
type vs. adenoid cystic carcinoma and
other types of infiltrating carcinoma,
88–93, *90–93*
medullary type, vs. atypical medullary
carcinoma vs. malignant lymphoma,
94–97, *96–97*
metaplastic type
vs. carcinosarcoma vs. pure sarcoma,
146–147, *147*
vs. fibromatosis vs. fibrosarcoma, 154–155,
155
vs. stromal proliferations, 98–101, *99–101*
mucinous (colloid) type, vs. mucocele-like
lesions vs. cystic hypersecretory carcinoma
vs. juvenile papillomatosis, 102–107,
104–107
Infiltrating, lobular
vs. LCIS and ALH in radial sclerosing lesions,
62–63, *63*
of classic type, vs. other patterns of infiltrating
lobular carcinoma, 108–112, *110–112*
vs. LCIS in sclerosing adenosis, 20–21, *21*
vs. sclerosing adenosis with marked ductular
attenuation, 12–13, *13*
Carcinosarcoma vs. metaplastic carcinoma vs. pure
sarcoma, 146–147, *147*
carcinoma with prominent spindle cell
metaplasia, *147*
cytokeratin immunoperoxidase, *147*
carcinoma with spindle cell metaplasia, *147*
carcinoma with squamous and spindle cell
metaplasia, *147*
metaplastic carcinoma, *147*
Collagenous spherulosis vs. cribriform ductal
carcinoma *in situ* and adenoid cystic
carcinoma, 52–53, *53*
adenoid cystic carcinoma, *53*

collagenous spherulosis, *53*
cribriform ductal carcinoma *in situ, 53*
Cribriform ductal carcinoma
in situ and adenoid cystic carcinoma vs.
collagenous spherulosis, 52–53, *53*
adenoid cystic carcinoma, *53*
collagenous spherulosis, *53*
cribriform ductal carcinoma *in situ, 53*
in situ vs. infiltrating cribriform carcinoma,
40–41, *41*
cribriform ductal carcinoma *in situ, 41*
infiltrating cribriform carcinoma, *41, 90*
infiltrating cribriform carcinoma vs. ductal
carcinoma *in situ* of cribriform type vs.
adenoid cystic carcinoma, 40–41, *41,*
88–93, *90–91, 93*
adenoid cystic carcinoma, *91*
ductal carcinoma *in situ*
cribriform, *91*
myoepithelium stained with actin, *90*
infiltrating cribriform carcinoma, *90,* 41
infiltrating duct carcinoma with stromal giant
cells, *93*
infiltrating vs. cribriform ductal carcinoma *in situ,*
40–41, *41*
cribriform ductal carcinoma *in situ, 41*
infiltrating cribriform carcinoma, *41*

D
Densities with smooth borders vs. densities with
spiculation, 168–169, *169*
circumscribed round density, *169*
colloid carcinoma, *169*
infiltrating ductal carcinoma, *169*
radial sclerosing lesion, *169*
spiculated density, linear calcifications, *169*
Ductal and lobular proliferations, 24–53
apocrine hyperplasia and atypical apocrine
hyperplasia vs. intraductal apocrine
carcinoma, 42–45, *43, 45*
apocrine hyperplasia, *43*
apocrine ductal carcinoma *in situ, 45*
atypical apocrine hyperplasia, *43*
papillary apocrine hyperplasia, *43*
clinical overview, 24
collagenous spherulosis vs. cribriform ductal
carcinoma *in situ* and adenoid cystic
carcinoma, 52–53, *53*
adenoid cystic carcinoma, *53*
collagenous spherulosis, *53*
cribriform ductal carcinoma *in situ, 53*
cribriform ductal carcinoma *in situ* vs. infiltrating
cribriform carcinoma, 40–41, *41*
cribriform ductal carcinoma *in situ, 41, 90*
infiltrating cribriform carcinoma, *41, 90*
ductal carcinoma *in situ*
lobular extension of vs. ductal extension of
lobular carcinoma *in situ,* 48–51, *49, 51*
ductal carcinoma *in situ* in hyperplasia, *51*
ductal carcinoma *in situ* in lobule, *49*
lobular carcinoma *in situ*
with duct extension, *51*
in hyperplasia, *51*
in pagetoid spread, *51*
low-grade vs. intermediate and high-grade ductal
carcinoma *in situ,* 36–39, *37, 39*
clear cell comedo ductal carcinoma *in situ, 39*
comedo ductal carcinoma *in situ, 37*
high-grade cribriform ductal carcinoma *in
situ, 37, 39*
high-grade micropapillary ductal carcinoma
in situ, 37
intermediate-grade cribriform ductal
carcinoma *in situ, 39*
low-grade cribriform ductal carcinoma *in
situ, 39*
low-grade micropapillary ductal carcinoma
in situ, 37

gross morphology, overview, 25
hyperplasia
usual, and atypical ductal hyperplasia vs. low-
grade ductal hyperplasia *in situ,* 30–35,
31–35
cribriform ductal carcinoma *in situ, 31*
intermediate grade, *31*
ductal carcinoma *in situ,* low grade, *32*
cribriform ductal carcinoma *in situ, 32*
fine needle aspiration, *32*
micropapillary ductal carcinoma *in situ, 34*
micropapillary usual hyperplasia, *33*
solid ductal carcinoma *in situ, 35*
solid usual hyperplasia, *35*
usual hyperplasia, *31, 32*
fine needle aspiration
usual vs. atypical ductal hyperplasia, 26–29,
27, 29
atypical ductal hyperplasia, *28*
usual hyperplasia, *27*
usual and atypical lobular hyperplasia vs.
lobular carcinoma *in situ,* 46–47, *47*
atypical lobular hyperplasia, *47*
lobular carcinoma *in situ, 47*
imaging, 24–25
overview, 24
Ductal carcinoma, infiltrating
vs. ductal carcinoma *in situ* in sclerosing
adenosis, 18–19, *19*
ductal carcinoma *in situ* in sclerosing adenosis,
19
infiltrating ductal carcinoma, *19*
vs. tubular carcinoma, 84–87, *85–87*
infiltrating ductal carcinoma, *85, 86*
apocrine type, *87*
fine needle aspiration, *87*
trapped ductules in radial scar, *85*
tubular carcinoma, *85, 86*
fine needle aspiration, *87*
tubular carcinoma with ductal carcinoma *in
situ, 85*
tubulolobular carcinoma, *87*
Ductal carcinoma associated with papilloma,
infiltrating, vs. papilloma with sclerotic
alterations, 74–75
papilloma(s) with sclerosis, *75*
sclerosed papilloma (ductal adenoma), *75*
Ductal carcinoma *in situ*
with central necrosis and calcification, *171, 172*
comedo type, *171*
cribriform, type, *172*
cribriform type vs. adenoid cystic carcinoma vs.
cribriform carcinoma, infiltrating, 88–93,
90–91, 93
infiltrating cribriform carcinoma, *90*
intermediate, and high-grade, vs. low-grade ductal
carcinoma *in situ,* 36–39, *37, 39*
clear cell comedo ductal carcinoma *in situ, 39*
comedo ductal carcinoma *in situ, 37*
high-grade cribriform ductal carcinoma *in situ,
37, 39*
high-grade micropapillary ductal carcinoma *in
situ, 37*
intermediate-grade cribriform ductal carcinoma
in situ, 39
low-grade cribriform ductal carcinoma *in situ,
39*
low-grade micropapillary ductal carcinoma *in
situ, 37*
lobular extension of, vs. ductal extension of lobular
carcinoma *in situ,* 48–51, *49, 51*
ductal carcinoma *in situ*
with lobular extension, *49, 51*
in hyperplasia, *49, 51*
lobular carcinoma *in situ*
with duct extension, *51*
in hyperplasia, *51*
in pagetoid spread, *51*

Ductal carcinoma *in situ* (contd.)
  low-grade
    vs. intermediate and high-grade ductal
        carcinoma *in situ*, 36–39, *37, 39*
      clear cell comedo ductal carcinoma *in situ*, *39*
      comedo ductal carcinoma *in situ*, *37*
      high-grade cribriform ductal carcinoma *in
          situ*, *37, 39*
      high-grade micropapillary ductal carcinoma
          in situ, *37*
      intermediate-grade cribriform ductal
          carcinoma *in situ*, *39*
      low-grade cribriform ductal carcinoma *in
          situ*, *39*
      low-grade micropapillary ductal carcinoma
          in situ, *37*
    vs. usual hyperplasia and atypical ductal
        hyperplasia, 30–35, *31–35*
      ductal carcinoma *in situ*, cribriform, 31, *32*
      ductal carcinoma *in situ*, low grade, 31, *32*
      ductal carcinoma *in situ*, micropapillary, *33,
          34*
      ductal carcinoma *in situ* solid, low grade, *35*
      micropapillary usual hyperplasia, *33*
      solid usual hyperplasia, *35*
      usual hyperplasia, *31*
    within radial sclerosing lesions vs. usual radial
        scars and infiltrating carcinoma, 58–61,
        59, 61
      atypical hyperplasia in sclerosing lesion, *59*
      ductal carcinoma *in situ* in sclerosing lesion, *61*
      infiltrating cribriform carcinoma, *61*
      radial sclerosing lesion, *59*
    in sclerosing adenosis vs. infiltrating ductal
        carcinoma, 18–19, *19*
      ductal carcinoma *in situ* in sclerosing adenosis,
          19
      infiltrating ductal carcinoma, *19*
Ductal extension of lobular carcinoma *in situ* vs.
    lobular extension of ductal carcinoma *in
    situ*, 48–51, *49, 51*
  ductal carcinoma *in situ* in lobule, *49*
  lobular carcinoma *in situ* in pagetoid spread, *51*
  lobular carcinoma *in situ* with duct extension, *51*
Ductal hyperplasia
  atypical, vs. usual hyperplasia, 26–29, *27, 29*
    ductal hyperplasia, atypical, *29*
    hyperplasia, usual, *27*
  atypical, and ductal carcinoma *in situ* in
      sclerosing adenosis vs. atypical lobular
      hyperplasia and lobular carcinoma *in situ*
      in sclerosing adenosis, 22–23, *23*
  ductal carcinoma *in situ* in sclerosing adenosis vs.
      lobular carcinoma *in situ* in sclerosing
      adenosis
    ductal carcinoma *in situ* in adenosis, *23*
    lobular carcinoma *in situ* in adenosis, 23

F
Fat necrosis vs. histiocytoid carcinoma vs. lipid-rich
    carcinoma, 158–159, *159*
  histiocytoid carcinoma with foamy cells, *159*
  lipid-rich carcinoma, *159*
Fibroadenoma of adult type, vs. low-grade phyllodes
    tumor, vs. juvenile fibroadenoma,
    136–137, *137*
  juvenile fibroadenoma, *137*
  phyllodes tumor, *137*
Fibroadenoma vs. low-grade phyllodes tumor,
    128–135, *130–135*
  Fibroadenoma
    with apocrine metaplasia, *131*
    with calcification, 170, *173*
    cellular fibroadenoma, *131, 135*
    ductal carcinoma *in situ* in fibroadenoma, *132*
    fibroadenoma phyllodes, *131, 135*
    with fibrocystic changes, *131*
    fine needle aspiration, *130*

intracanalicular, *130, 135*
lobular carcinoma *in situ* in, *132*
mixed pattern, *130*
pericanalicular, *130*
with usual epithelial hyperplasia
  phyllodes tumor
    core needle biopsy, *133*
    with fibrocystic changes, *133*
    fine needle aspiration, *133*
    with liposarcomatous stroma, *134*
    lobular carcinoma *in situ* in
    low grade, *135*
    with spindle cell (fibrosarcomatous) stroma, *134*
Fibroadenoma with infiltrating carcinoma vs.
    fibroadenoma with superimposed
    sclerosing adenosis, 138–139, *139*
  adenosis in fibroadenoma, *139*
  infiltrating lobular carcinoma in fibroadenoma,
      139
  infiltrating tubular carcinoma in fibroadenoma,
      139
  sclerosing adenosis with attenuated ductules in
      fibroadenoma, *139*
Fibromatosis vs. fibrosarcoma vs. metaplastic
    carcinoma, 154–155, *155*
  carcinoma with prominent spindle cell
      metaplasia, *155*
  fibromatosis, *155*
  fibrosarcoma, *155*
Fibrosarcoma vs. metaplastic carcinoma vs.
    fibromatosis, 154–155, *155*
Florid papillomatosis of nipple vs. well-differentiated
    carcinoma vs. syringomatous adenoma,
    114–119, *115–117, 119*
  cribriform ductal carcinoma *in situ*, *117*
  nipple duct adenoma, *115–117, 119*
  papillary carcinoma, *116*
  syringomatous adenoma, *119*
  tubular carcinoma, *117*

G
Giant cells, stromal infiltrating carcinoma, 89, *93*
Granular cell tumor vs. histiocytoid carcinoma,
    156–157, *157*
  granular cell tumor, *157*
  histiocytoid carcinoma with granular cells
      (myoblastomatoid carcinoma), *157*

H
Histiocytoid carcinoma
  vs. granular cell tumor, 156–157, *157*
    granular cell tumor, *157*
    histiocytoid carcinoma with granular cells
        (myoblastomatoid carcinoma), *157*
  vs. lipid-rich carcinoma vs. fat necrosis, 158–159,
      159
    fat necrosis, *159*
    histiocytoid carcinoma with foamy cells, *159*
    lipid-rich carcinoma, *159*
Hyperplasia
  usual and atypical ductal hyperplasia vs. low-
      grade ductal carcinoma *in situ*, 30–35,
      31–35
    cribriform ductal carcinoma *in situ*, *31, 32*
    ductal carcinoma *in situ*, low grade, *32*
    micropapillary ductal carcinoma *in situ*, *33, 34*
    micropapillary usual hyperplasia, *33, 35*
    solid ductal carcinoma *in situ*, low grade, *35*
    solid usual hyperplasia, *35*
    usual hyperplasia, *31, 32*
  usual vs. atypical ductal hyperplasia, 26–29, *27,
      29*
    ductal hyperplasia, atypical, *28*
    hyperplasia, usual, *27*

I
Infiltrating carcinoma, special types, 83–112
  clinical overview, 83

gross morphology, overview, 83
imaging, 83
vs. lobular carcinoma *in situ* and atypical lobular
    hyperplasia in radial sclerosing lesions,
    62–63, *63*
  atypical hyperplasia in sclerosing lesion, *63*
  invasive lobular carcinoma, *63*
  lobular neoplasia
    in adenosis, *63*
    in sclerosing lesion, *63*
  radial sclerosing lesion, *63*
  sclerosing lesion with apocrine cells, *63*
overview, 83
vs. postbiopsy and traumatic alterations in *in situ*
    carcinoma, 64–65, *65*
  posttraumatic pseudoinvasion, *65*
vs. radial sclerosing lesions, 55–57, *56–57*
  radial sclerosing lesion, *56, 57*
  tubular carcinoma, *57*
  with low-grade ductal carcinoma *in situ*, *57*
Infiltrating lobular carcinoma of classical type vs.
    other patterns of infiltrating lobular
    carcinoma, 108–112, *110–112*
Infiltrating papillary carcinoma vs. non-infiltrating
    papillary carcinoma with
    pseudoinfiltration, 81, *81*
  non-infiltrating papillary carcinoma with
      pseudoinfiltration, *81*
  papillary carcinoma with focal stromal infiltration,
      81
Intraductal apocrine carcinoma vs. apocrine
    hyperplasia and atypical apocrine
    hyperplasia, 42–45, *43, 45*
  apocrine hyperplasia, *43*
  apocrine ductal carcinoma *in situ*, *45*
  atypical apocrine hyperplasia, *43*
  papillary apocrine hyperplasia, *43*
Intraductal (non-infiltrating) papillary carcinoma vs.
    papilloma, 69–73, *70–73*
  duct papilloma, *70, 71*
  FNA cell block, *71*
  intracystic papillary carcinoma with adjacent
      ductal carcinoma *in situ*, *73*
  multiple duct papillomas, *70*
  papillary carcinoma, *72, 73*
  FNA cell block, *73*
  papillary carcinoma actin immunoperoxidase, *73*
  papillary lesion, *71, 73*
  FNA smear, *71, 73*
  solitary duct papilloma, *70*

J
Juvenile fibroadenoma vs. fibroadenoma of adult
    type vs. low-grade phyllodes tumor,
    136–137, *137*
  fibroadenoma, *137*
  juvenile fibroadenoma, *137*
  phyllodes tumor, *137*

L
Lobular and ductal proliferations, 24–53
  apocrine hyperplasia and atypical apocrine
      hyperplasia vs. intraductal apocrine
      carcinoma, 42–45, *43, 45*
    apocrine hyperplasia, *43*
    apocrine ductal carcinoma *in situ*, *45*
    atypical apocrine hyperplasia, *43*
    papillary apocrine hyperplasia, *43*
  clinical overview, 24
  collagenous spherulosis vs. cribriform ductal
      carcinoma *in situ* and adenoid cystic
      carcinoma, 52–53, *53*
    adenoid cystic carcinoma, *53*
    collagenous spherulosis, *53*
    cribriform ductal carcinoma *in situ*, *53*
  cribriform ductal carcinoma *in situ* vs. infiltrating
      cribriform carcinoma, 40–41, *41, 90*
    cribriform ductal carcinoma *in situ*, *41, 90*

Lobular, and ductal proliferation (contd.)
    infiltrating cribriform carcinoma, 41, 90
  ductal carcinoma in situ, low-grade, vs.
      intermediate and high-grade ductal
      carcinoma in situ, 36–39, 37, 39
    clear cell comedo ductal carcinoma in situ, 39
    comedo ductal carcinoma in situ, 37
    high-grade cribriform ductal carcinoma in situ,
      37, 39
    high-grade micropapillary ductal carcinoma in
      situ, 37
    intermediate-grade cribriform ductal carcinoma
      in situ, 39
    low-grade cribriform ductal carcinoma in situ,
      39
    low-grade micropapillary ductal carcinoma in
      situ, 37
  ductal carcinoma in situ, lobular extension of, vs.
      ductal extension of lobular carcinoma in
      situ, 48–51, 49, 51
    ductal carcinoma in situ in hyperplasia, 51
    ductal carcinoma in situ in lobule, 49
    lobular carcinoma in situ
      with duct extension, 51
      in hyperplasia, 51
      in pagetoid spread, 51
  gross morphology, overview, 25
  hyperplasia
    usual, and atypical ductal hyperplasia vs. low-
      grade ductal carcinoma in situ, 30–35,
      31–35
      cribriform ductal carcinoma in situ, 31, 32
      fine needle aspiration, 32
      ductal carcinoma in situ, low grade, 32
      micropapillary ductal carcinoma in situ, 33,
        34
      micropapillary usual hyperplasia, 33
      solid ductal carcinoma in situ
        low grade, 35
      solid usual hyperplasia, 35
      usual hyperplasia, 31
      fine needle aspiration
    usual vs. atypical ductal hyperplasia, 26–29,
      27, 29
      ductal hyperplasia, atypical, 28
      hyperplasia, usual, 27
  imaging, 24–25
  lobular hyperplasia, usual
    and atypical lobular hyperplasia vs. lobular
      carcinoma in situ, 46–47, 47
      atypical lobular hyperplasia, 47
      lobular carcinoma in situ, 47
  overview, 24
Lobular carcinoma
  of classical type, infiltrating, vs. other patterns of
      infiltrating lobular carcinoma, 108–112,
      110–112
    infiltrating lobular carcinoma, 110–112
      alveolar pattern, 111
      with lobular carcinoma in situ, 111
      with mucin vacuoles, 111
      with pleomorphic nuclei, 112
  infiltrating, vs. sclerosing adenosis with marked
      ductular attenuation, 12–13, 13
    infiltrating lobular carcinoma, 13
    sclerosing adenosis with attenuated ductules, 13
  in situ vs. usual lobular hyperplasia and atypical
      lobular hyperplasia, 46–47, 47
    atypical lobular hyperplasia, 47
    lobular carcinoma in situ, 47
  in situ and atypical lobular hyperplasia in radial
      sclerosing lesions vs. infiltrating carcinoma,
      62–63, 63
    atypical hyperplasia, in sclerosing lesion, 63
    infiltrating lobular carcinoma, 63
    lobular neoplasia
      in adenosis, 63
      in sclerosing lesion, 63

    radial sclerosing lesion, 63
    sclerosing lesion with apocrine cells, 63
  in situ in sclerosing adenosis vs. infiltrating
      lobular carcinoma, 20–21, 21
    infiltrating lobular carcinoma, 21
    lobular carcinoma in situ in adenosis, 21
  vs lobular carcinoma in situ in sclerosing
      adenosis, 20–21, 21
    infiltrating lobular carcinoma, 21
    lobular carcinoma in situ
      in sclerosing adenosis, 21
  metastatic
    vs. malignant lymphoma, axillary lymph node,
      165, 165
      lymph node
        diffuse lymphoma, large cell type, 165
        metastatic lobular carcinoma, diffuse
          pattern, 165
    vs. sinus histiocytosis, axillary lymph node,
      164, 164
      lymph node
        metastatic lobular carcinoma, sinus catarrh
          pattern, 164
        sinus histiocytosis, 164
Lobular hyperplasia
  lobular carcinoma in situ and atypical lobular
      hyperplasia in sclerosing adenosis, vs.
      atypical ductal hyperplasia and ductal
      carcinoma in situ in sclerosing adenosis,
      22–23, 23
    ductal carcinoma in situ in adenosis, 23
    lobular carcinoma in situ in adenosis, 23
  usual and atypical lobular hyperplasia vs. lobular
      carcinoma in situ, 46–47, 47
    atypical lobular hyperplasia, 47
    lobular carcinoma in situ, 47
Lymph nodes. See also axillary lymph node lesions
Lymphoma, malignant, axillary lymph nodes, vs.
      metastatic lobular carcinoma, 165, 165
  lymph node
    diffuse lymphoma, large cell type, 165
    metastatic lobular carcinoma, diffuse pattern,
      165
Lymphoma, malignant, vs. medullary carcinoma,
      94–97, 96, 97

M
Mammary stroma, pseudoangiomatous hyperplasia
      of, vs. angiosarcoma, 148–149, 149
Medullary carcinoma vs. atypical medullary
      carcinoma vs. malignant lymphoma,
      94–97, 96–97
  atypical medullary carcinoma, 96
  malignant lymphoma, 97
  medullary carcinoma, 97
Mesenchymal and biphasic proliferations
  angiosarcoma, poorly differentiated, vs. other
      spindle cell tumors, 153, 153
    amelanotic spindle cell melanoma, 153
    angiosarcoma, poorly differentiated, 153
    carcinoma with prominent spindle cell
      metaplasia, 153
    fibrosarcoma, 153
  carcinosarcoma vs. metaplastic carcinoma vs.
      pure sarcoma, 146–147, 147
    carcinoma with prominent spindle cell
      metaplasia, cytokeratin immunoperoxidase,
      147
    carcinoma with spindle cell metaplasia, 147
    carcinoma with squamous and spindle cell
      metaplasia, 147
    metaplastic carcinoma, 147
  clinical overview, 125–126
  fat necrosis vs. histiocytoid carcinoma vs. lipid-
      rich carcinoma, 158–159, 159
    fat necrosis, 159
    histiocytoid carcinoma with foamy cells, 159
    lipid-rich carcinoma, 159

fibroadenoma vs. low-grade phyllodes tumor,
    128–135, 130–135
  cellular fibroadenoma, 131, 135
  ductal carcinoma in situ in fibroadenoma,
    132
  fibroadenoma
    with apocrine metaplasia, 131
    with fibrocystic changes, 131
    fine needle aspiration, 130
    intracanalicular pattern, 130
    mixed pattern, 130
    pericanalicular pattern, 130
    with usual epithelial hyperplasia, 131
  fibroadenoma phyllodes, 131, 135
  liposarcomatous stroma with osseous
    metaplasia, phyllodes tumor, 134
  lobular carcinoma in situ
    in fibroadenoma, 132
    in phyllodes tumor, 134
  phyllodes tumor, 132, 133
    core needle biopsy, 133
    with fibrocystic changes, 133
    fine needle aspiration, 133
    with liposarcomatous stroma, 134
    low grade, 135
    with spindle cell (fibrosarcomatous) stroma,
      134
fibroadenoma with superimposed sclerosing
    adenosis vs. fibroadenoma with infiltrating
    carcinoma, 138–139, 139
  adenosis in fibroadenoma, 139
  infiltrating lobular carcinoma in fibroadenoma,
    139
  infiltrating tubular carcinoma in fibroadenoma,
    139
  sclerosing adenosis with attenuated ductules in
    fibroadenoma, 139
fibromatosis vs. fibrosarcoma vs. metaplastic
    carcinoma, 154–155, 155
  carcinoma with prominent spindle cell
    metaplasia, 155
  fibromatosis, 155
  fibrosarcoma, 155
granular cell tumor vs. histiocytoid carcinoma,
    156–157, 157
  granular cell tumor, 157
  histiocytoid carcinoma with granular cells
    (myoblastomatoid carcinoma), 157
gross morphology, overview, 127
imaging, 126
juvenile fibroadenoma vs. fibroadenoma of adult
    type vs. low-grade phyllodes tumor,
    136–137, 137
  fibroadenoma, 137
  juvenile fibroadenoma, 137
  phyllodes tumor, 137
overview, 124–126
periductal stromal sarcoma vs. phyllodes tumor
    vs. pure sarcoma, 144–145, 145
  periductal stromal sarcoma, 145
  phyllodes tumor, 145
  pure spindle cell sarcoma, 145
phyllodes tumor
  high-grade, with sarcomatous overgrowth vs.
      pure sarcoma, 142–143, 143
    phyllodes tumor, high grade
      with fibrosarcomatous overgrowth, 143
      with liposarcomatous overgrowth, 143
  low-grade, vs. high-grade (malignant) phyllodes
      tumor, 140–141, 141
    phyllodes tumor
      high grade, 141
      low grade, 141
pseudoangiomatous hyperplasia of mammary
    stroma vs. angiosarcoma, 148–149, 149
  angiosarcoma, 149
  pseudoangiomatous hyperplasia of mammary
    stroma, 149

Mesenchymal and biphasic proliferations *(contd.)*
vascular proliferations, benign, vs. angiosarcoma, 150–152, *152*
angiolipoma, *152*
angiosarcoma, 151, *152*
hemangioma, 151, *152*
intravascular papillary endothelial hyperplasia, *152*
Metaplastic carcinoma
vs. carcinosarcoma vs. pure sarcoma, 146–147, *147*
carcinoma with prominent spindle cell metaplasia, cytokeratin immunoperoxidase, *147*
carcinoma with spindle cell metaplasia, *147*
carcinoma with squamous and spindle cell metaplastic, *147*
metaplastic carcinoma, *147*
vs. fibrosarcoma, vs. fibromatosis, 154–155, *155*
vs. stromal proliferations, 98–101, *99, 101*
Carcinoma with squamous metaplasia, FNA, *99*
metaplastic carcinoma, *99, 101*
cytokeratin immunoperoxidase, *101*
metaplastic carcinoma with angiosarcoma-like areas, *99*
metaplastic carcinoma with cartilaginous matrix, *101*
carcinoma with squamous metaplasia, *99*
phyllodes tumor, *101*
Metastatic tumors, axillary lymph nodes, vs. capsular nevus cell aggregates and nodal glandular inclusions, 162–163, *163*
lymph nodes
benign glandular inclusions, *163*
capsular nevus cell aggregates, *163*
metastatic ductal carcinoma, *163*
metastatic lobular carcinoma, *163*
Microglandular adenosis vs. tubular carcinoma, 14–15, *15*
microglandular adenosis, *15*
tubular carcinoma, *15*
Mucinous (colloid) carcinoma vs. mucocele-like lesions vs. cystic hypersecretory carcinoma vs. juvenile papillomatosis, 102–107, *104–105, 107*
cystic hypersecretory carcinoma, *107*
juvenile papillomatosis, *107*
mucinous carcinoma, *104, 169*
fine needle aspiration, *105*
mucinous cerinoma with ductal carcinoma *in situ*, *104*
mucocele-like lesion, *105*
Mucocele-like lesions, vs. cystic hypersecretory carcinoma, vs. juvenile papillomatosis, vs. mucinous (colloid) carcinoma, 102–107, *104–105, 107*
cystic hypersecretory carcinoma, *107*
juvenile papillomatosis, *107*
mucinous carcinoma, *104*
with ductal carcinoma *in situ*, *104*
fine needle aspiration, *105*
mucocele-like lesion, *105*
Myoblastomatoid carcinoma, 57, *157*

N

Nipple disorders, 113–123
clinical overview, 113
duct adenoma (florid papillomatosis of nipple) vs. well-differentiated carcinoma vs. syringomatous adenoma, 114–119, *115–117, 119*
cribriform ductal carcinoma *in situ*, *117*
nipple duct adenoma, *115–117, 119*
papillary carcinoma, *116*
syringomatous adenoma, *119*
tubular carcinoma, *117*
overview, 113

Paget disease of nipple vs. cutaneous tumors, 120–123, *121–123*
Bowen disease, *123*
ductal carcinoma *in situ* in Paget disease, *121*
malignant melanoma, *121, 122*
Paget disease, *121, 122, 123*
EMA immunoperoxidase, *122*
low molecular weight cytokeratin immunoperoxidase, *122*

P

Paget disease of nipple vs. cutaneous tumors, 120–123, *121–123*
Bowen disease, *123*
ductal carcinoma *in situ* in Paget disease, *121*
malignant melanoma, *122*
Paget disease, *121–123*
EMA immunoperoxidase, *122*
low molecular weight cytokeratin immunoperoxidase, *122*
Papillary lesions, 66–81
atypical epithelial hyperplasia in papilloma (atypical papilloma) vs. non-infiltrating (intraductal) carcinoma arising in papilloma, 80, *80*
clinical overview, 66–67
gross morphology, overview, 67–68
imaging, 67
infiltrating papillary carcinoma vs. non-infiltrating papillary carcinoma with pseudoinfiltration, 81, *81*
non-infiltrating papillary carcinoma with pseudoinfiltration, *81*
papillary carcinoma with focal stromal invasion, *81*
overview, 66
papilloma vs. intraductal (non-infiltrating) papillary carcinoma, 69–73, *70–73*
duct papilloma, *70, 71*
FNA cell block, *71*
FNA smear, *71, 73*
intracystic papillary carcinoma with adjacent ductal carcinoma *in situ*, *73*
solitary duct papilloma, *70*
multiple duct papillomas, *70*
papillary carcinoma, *72, 73*
actin immunoperoxidase, *73*
CEA immunoperoxidase, *73*
FNA cell block, *73*
intracystic, *73*
papilloma with metaplastic alterations vs. carcinoma, 76–79, *77, 79*
apocrine metaplasia
with atypical hyperplasia in papilloma, *79*
FNA cell block, *77*
FNA smear, *77*
with hyperplasia in papilloma, *77, 79*
in papilloma, *77*
in sclerosing papilloma, *79*
squamous metaplasia
in papilloma, *79*
papilloma with sclerotic alterations vs. infiltrating ductal carcinoma associated with papilloma, 74–75
papilloma with sclerosis, *75*
sclerosed papilloma (ductal adenoma), *75*
Papilloma, non-infiltrating (intraductal) carcinoma arising in, vs. atypical epithelial hyperplasia in papilloma (atypical papilloma), 80, *80*
Papillomatosis of nipple, florid, vs. well-differentiated carcinoma vs. syringomatous adenoma, 114–119, *115–117, 119*
cribriform ductal carcinoma *in situ*, *117*
nipple duct adenoma, *115–117, 119*
papillary carcinoma, *116*
syringomatous adenoma, *119*
tubular carcinoma, *117*

Papilloma vs. intraductal (non-infiltrating) papillary carcinoma, 69–73, *70–73*
duct papilloma, *70, 71*
FNA cell block, *71*
intracystic papillary carcinoma with adjacent ductal carcinoma *in situ*, *73*
solitary duct papilloma, *70*
multiple duct papillomas, *70*
papillary carcinoma, *72, 73*
actin immunoperoxidase, *73*
CEA immunoperoxidase, *73*
FNA cell block, *73*
intracystic, *73*
papillary lesion
FNA smear, *71, 73*
Papilloma with metaplastic alterations vs. carcinoma, 76–79, *77, 79*
apocrine metaplasia
with atypical hyperplasia in papilloma, *79*
FNA cell block, *77*
FNA smear, *77*
with hyperplasia in papilloma, *77, 79*
in papilloma, *77*
in sclerosing papilloma, *79*
squamous metaplasia
in infarcted papilloma, *79*
in papilloma, *79*
Papilloma with sclerotic alterations vs. infiltrating ductal carcinoma associated with papilloma, 74–75
papilloma(s) with sclerosis, *75*
sclerosed papilloma (ductal adenoma), *75*
Periductal stromal sarcoma vs. phyllodes tumor vs. pure sarcoma, 144–145, *145*
periductal stromal sarcoma, *145*
phyllodes tumor, *145*
pure spindle cell sarcoma, *145*
Perineural invasion by infiltrating carcinoma, vs. sclerosing adenosis, perineural space extension in, 6–7, *7*
perineural extension, sclerosing adenosis, *7*
perineural invasion, infiltrating carcinoma, *7*
Phyllodes tumor
high-grade
vs. phyllodes tumor, low-grade, 140–141, *141*
phyllodes tumor
high grade, *141*
low grade, *141*
with sarcomatous overgrowth vs. pure sarcoma, 142–143, *143*
phyllodes tumor, high grade
with fibrosarcomatous stromal overgrowth, *143*
with liposarcomatous stromal overgrowth, *143*
low-grade
vs. fibroadenoma, 128–135, *130–135*
with apocrine metaplasia, *131*
cellular fibroadenoma, *131, 135*
ductal carcinoma *in situ* in fibroadenoma, *132*
fibroadenoma
fine needle aspiration, *130*
intracanalicular pattern, *130, 135*
mixed pattern, *130*
pericanalicular pattern, *130*
fibroadenoma phyllodes, *131, 135*
with fibrocystic changes, *131*
lobular carcinoma *in situ*
in fibroadenoma, *132*
in phyllodes tumor, *134*
phyllodes tumor, *132, 133*
core needle biopsy, *133*
with fibrocystic changes, *133*
fine needle aspiration, *133*
with liposarcomatous stroma, *134*
low grade, *135*
with spindle cell (fibrosarcomatous) stroma, *134*

Phyllodes tumor (contd.)
  with usual epithelial hyperplasia, 131
  vs. high-grade phyllodes tumor, 140–141, 141
    phyllodes tumor
      high grade, 141
      low grade, 141
  vs. pure sarcoma vs. periductal stromal sarcoma,
      144–145, 145
    periductal stromal sarcoma, 145
    phyllodes tumor, 145
    pure spindle cell sarcoma, 145
Postbiopsy, traumatic alterations, in situ carcinoma
      vs. infiltrating carcinoma, 64–65, 65
  posttraumatic pseudoinvasion, 65
Pseudoangiomatous hyperplasia of mammary stroma
      vs. angiosarcoma, 148–149, 149
    angiosarcoma, 149
    pseudoangiomatous hyperplasia of mammary
      stroma, 149

R
Radial scars
  complex sclerosing lesions vs. sclerosing
      adenosis, 16–17, 17
    radial scar, 17
    sclerosing adenosis, 17
  infiltrating carcinoma, vs. ductal carcinoma in situ
      within radial sclerosing lesions, 58–61, 59,
      61
    atypical hyperplasia in sclerosing lesion, 59
    ductal carcinoma in situ in sclerosing lesion, 61
    infiltrating cribriform carcinoma, 61
    radial sclerosing lesion, 59
  radial sclerosing lesions, and complex sclerosing
      lesions, 54–65
    gross morphology, overview, 54
    imaging, 54
    overview, 54
Radial sclerosing lesions vs. infiltrating carcinoma,
      55–57, 56–57
    radial sclerosing lesion, 56, 57
    tubular carcinoma, 57
    with low-grade ductal carcinoma in situ, 57
Radiographs, specimen, 167–173
  calcifications, highly suspicious vs. calcifications
      of intermediate concern, 170–173,
      171–173
    adenosis with calcifications, 173
    clustered calcification, 169, 171–173
    clustered cysts
      with calcium oxalate crystals, polarized,
        171
      unpolarized, 171
    ductal carcinoma in situ
      with central necrosis and calcification, 171,
        172
      comedo type, 171
      cribriform, 172
      fibroadenoma with calcifications, 173
      linear, casting calcifications, 171
  densities with smooth borders vs. densities with
      spiculation, 168–169, 169
    circumscribed round density, 169
    colloid carcinoma, 169
    infiltrating ductal carcinoma, 169

    radial sclerosing lesion, 169
    spiculated density, linear calcifications, 169
  overview, 167

S
Sarcoma. See also biphasic and mesenchymal
      proliferations
  Angiosarcoma
    vs. benign vascular proliferations, 150–151,
        151
    vs. pseudoangiomatous hyperplasia of
        mammary stroma, 148–149, 149
    poorly differentiated, vs. other malignant
        spindle cell tumors, 153, 153
  periductal stromal, vs. phyllodes tumor, vs. pure
      sarcoma, 144–145, 145
  pure, vs. phyllodes tumor, high grade, with
      sarcomatous overgrowth, 142–143, 143
  pure, vs. phyllodes tumor, vs. periductal stromal
      sarcoma, 144–145, 145
  pure, vs. carcinosarcoma, vs. metaplastic
      carcinoma, 146–147, 147
Sclerosing adenosis
  apocrine alterations, non neoplastic in, vs.
      apocrine carcinoma, 8–11, 9, 11
    apocrine ductal carcinoma in situ in sclerosing
        adenosis, 19, 11
    apocrine hyperplasia in sclerosing adenosis,
        atypical, 9
    apocrine metaplasia in sclerosing adenosis, 9, 11
        atypical, 11
    infiltrating apocrine carcinoma, 11
  with marked ductular attenuation vs. infiltrating
      lobular carcinoma, 12–13, 13
    infiltrating lobular carcinoma, 13
    sclerosing adenosis with attenuated ductules,
        13
  perineural space extension in vs. perineural
      invasion by infiltrating carcinoma, 6–7, 7
    perineural extension, sclerosing adenosis, 7
    perineural invasion, infiltrating carcinoma, 7
  vs. radial scars and complex sclerosing lesions,
      16–17, 17
    radial scar, 17
    sclerosing adenosis, 17
  vs. tubular carcinoma, 2–5, 3, 5
    adenosis, 5
    sclerosing adenosis, 3, 5
    tubular carcinoma, 5
Sinus histiocytosis, vs. metastatic lobular carcinoma
      in axillary lymph nodes, 164, 164
    metastatic lobular carcinoma, sinus catarrh
        pattern, 164
    sinus histiocytosis, 164
Specimen radiographs, 167–173
  calcifications, highly suspicious vs. calcifications
      of intermediate concern, 170–173,
      171–173
    adenosis with calcifications, 169, 173
    clustered calcifications, 171–173
    clustered cysts
      with calcium oxalate crystals, polarized,
        171
      unpolarized, 171
    ductal carcinoma in situ

    with central necrosis and calcification, 171,
        172
      comedo type, 171
      cribriform, 172
      fibroadenoma with calcification, 173
      linear, casting calcification, 171
  densities with smooth borders vs. densities with
      spiculation, 168–169, 169
    circumscribed round density, 169
    colloid carcinoma, 169
    infiltrating ductal carcinoma, 169
    radial sclerosing lesion, 169
    spiculated density, linear calcifications, 169
  overview, 167
Spindle cell tumors vs. angiosarcoma, poorly
      differentiated, 153, 153
    amelanotic spindle cell melanoma, 153
    angiosarcoma, poorly differentiated, 153
    carcinoma with prominent spindle cell
        metaplasia, 153
    fibrosarcoma, 153
Syringomatous adenoma, nipple, vs. well-
      differentiated carcinoma, vs. nipple duct
      adenoma (florid papillomatosis of nipple),
      114–119, 115–117, 119
    cribriform ductal carcinoma in situ, 117
    nipple duct adenoma, 115–117, 119
    papillary carcinoma, 116
    syringomatous adenoma, 119
    tubular carcinoma, 117

T
Traumatic alterations, postbiopsy, in situ carcinoma
      vs. infiltrating carcinoma, 64–65, 65
  posttraumatic pseudoinvasion, 65
Tubular carcinoma
  vs. microglandular adenosis, 14–15, 15
    microglandular adenosis, 15
    tubular carcinoma, 15
  vs. other types of infiltrating ductal carcinoma,
      84–87, 85–87
    infiltrating ductal carcinoma, 85, 86
    infiltrating ductal carcinoma
      apocrine type, 87
      fine needle aspiration, 87
      trapped ductules in radial scar, 85
    tubular carcinoma, 85, 86
      fine needle aspiration, 87
    tubular carcinoma with ductal carcinoma in
        situ, 85
    tubulolobular carcinoma, 87
  vs. sclerosing adenosis, 2–5, 3, 5
    adenosis, 5
    sclerosing adenosis, 3, 5
    tubular carcinoma, 5

V
Vascular proliferations, benign, vs. angiosarcoma,
      150–152, 152
    angiolipoma, 152
    angiosarcoma, 151, 152
    hemangioma, 151, 152
    intravascular papillary endothelial hyperplasia,
        152

ISBN 0-89640-314-9